KRISHNAM

in His Own Words

Asana • Pranayama • Meditation
Mantra • Ritual • Ayurveda

A. G. MOHAN

&

DR. GANESH MOHAN

ISBN-13 (International Edition): 978-981-18-5942-7

Publisher: Svastha Yoga

Contents

Introduction

Krishnamacharya as our guru

I met my guru Sri Krishnamacharya in 1971 and began my yoga studies with him that same year. I spent 18+ years studying with him personally, until his passing in 1989.

Krishnamacharya was an extraordinary person and a yogi of unique knowledge and practice. Hopefully, not much needs to be said to introduce him to the audience of this book. He received less acclaim than he deserved in his lifetime. However, as is often the case with great people in history, he is now widely acknowledged as one of the foremost yoga masters of the last century.

When I had the great fortune of joining as a student of Krishnamacharya, I was only 25 years old. I had a burning desire to pursue a spiritual path and yoga was my way to that. He was like a sage from the days of old; I had no hesitation in following him with deep trust.

Indra, my wife, has been my steadfast companion in this journey of learning and teaching yoga. My daughter Nitya and my son Ganesh, a medical doctor, have spent their early lives under the wisdom of Krishnamacharya's direction and have continued on that path later.

The word "guru" means "one who removes darkness." There are two types of gurus—one who sheds light on our material life and the one who gives us light in our spiritual path. Krishnamacharya was not one to interfere in the worldly life of his students. However, he was always keen on ensuring that dharma (ethics) and the practices of yoga should grow.

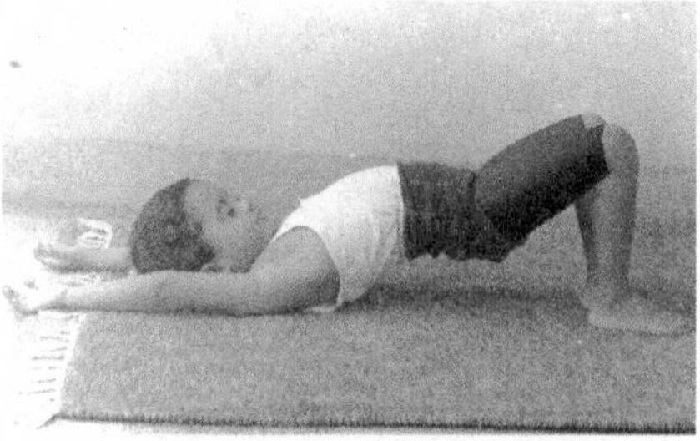
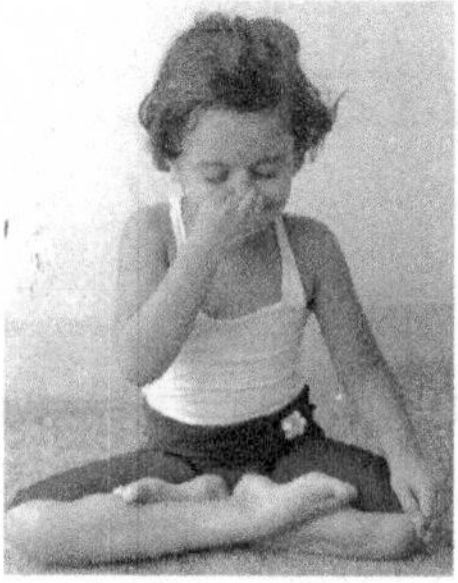

Nitya at 4 years (1977)

As the years passed, he was certain of my commitment to yoga and my trust in him. Therefore, while not getting into the material affairs of my life, he gave my whole family guidance on their path of yoga and wellbeing.

Regarding children and yoga, his view was that samskāra-s, our patterns, are vital. So, the earlier we start, the better. He gave Indra guidance on mudrā-s and chanting even during her pregnancy. Indra and I introduced Nitya to asanas when she was just 4 years old upon his suggestion. In 1977, he said, "If your daughter is old enough to eat by herself, you can start teaching her some simple asanas."

We followed the same advice with Ganesh too, having him practice asanas as a child. Since Indra and I were practicing every day, it was normal for them to follow us. This too was one of Krishnamacharya's important guidelines: we should lead children on the path of yoga by being an example as adults and parents.

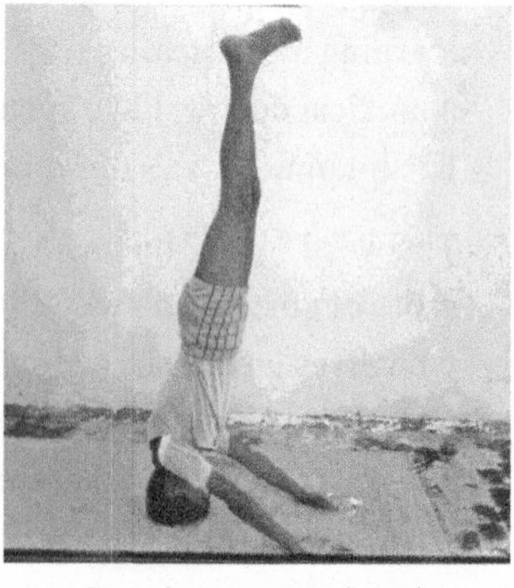

Ganesh at 10 years (1989)

He was of the view that women could also do Vedic chanting. This was a break from the orthodoxy of that time. Because of this, I started teaching Nitya Vedic chanting when she was just 4 years old. She had an excellent memory and good diction. As a child, Nitya did Vedic chanting at a traditional event where Krishnamacharya was present. He remarked to me afterwards, "Her pronunciation is good." This was an exceptional blessing. He was a strict taskmaster on the topic of accurate Vedic chanting, and to receive praise from him on that skill was a true rarity. She recorded an audio cassette on Vedic chanting, and also inaugurated the European Union of Yoga conference in Switzerland in 1983 with Vedic chanting, with Krishnamacharya's blessings.

Naturally, we taught Ganesh also Vedic chanting from when he was a child. It is traditional to start young boys chanting only after a sacred thread ritual is held. This is usually done after the child is a little older. However, Krishnamacharya told me, "Start teaching your son Vedic chanting as early as possible, even before these rituals can be done. The samskara-s are important."

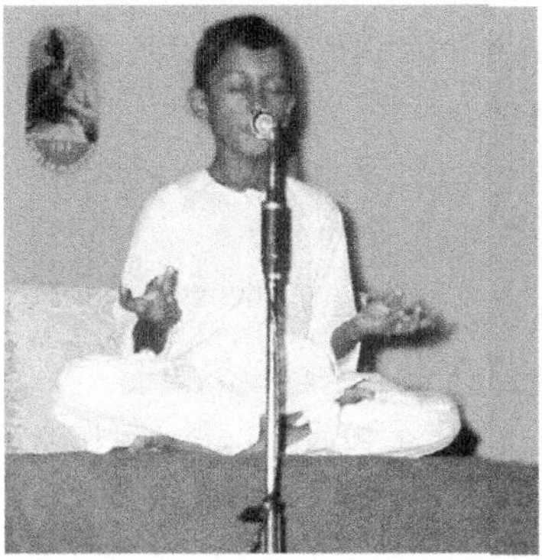
Ganesh demonstrating ritual (1988)

During Krishnamacharya's centenary celebrations in 1988, I delivered a lecture on the Vedic ritual of sandhyāvandana. To help with this presentation, I had Ganesh demonstrate the rituals and mantras as I spoke about them. I taught him the rituals first, then I took him to Krishnamacharya and had him demonstrate them in front of the master, to receive his approval. He was very pleased and then told me, "Teach your son everything you have learned. It should be passed on. He will do well."

He also told me that I should make my children learn Sanskrit early so that they would be able to read the traditional texts later.

Therefore, we had Nitya and Ganesh learn Sanskrit alongside their modern schooling.

Krishnamacharya has been the guiding light of our family.

Spreading the master's teachings

Krishnamacharya's lifelong wish was that yoga should spread widely. "Yoga propaganda" was the quaint term he used. He was always quick to add that *sound* yoga should be propagated. Unsound teachings, he would say, bring a bad name to yoga and to the yoga teacher.

As much as I have spent my adult lifetime studying and practicing yoga, I have also devoted my life to propagating its teachings—in keeping with the wishes of my master. We have worked together as a family for decades to spread the message of Krishnamacharya's teachings.

My formal efforts to spread the master's teachings began 45+ years ago. From 1975-1988, I served in many roles: trying to start a yoga magazine, planning for the institution of the Krishnamacharya Yoga Mandiram, serving as its honorary secretary, then the Associate Director of the KYM Institute of Yoga Studies when it was launched.

In 1988, I was the convenor of Krishnamacharya's centenary celebrations. The master passed away in 1989. From that time the next phase of my yoga journey commenced.

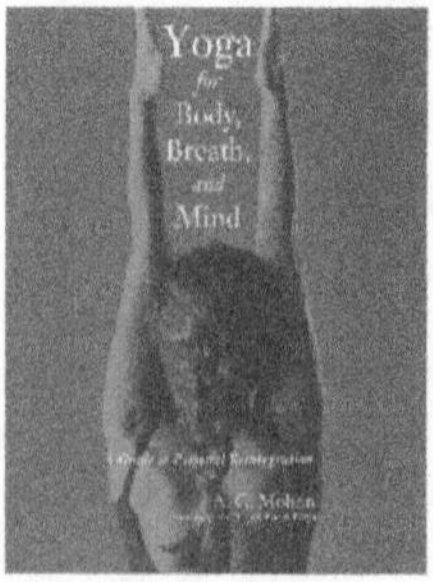

In 1993, my first book, *Yoga for Body, Breath, and Mind,* was published. It was dedicated to Sri Krishnamacharya. The goal of this book was to present yoga in a modern way while remaining faithful to the master's teachings as I understood it at that time.

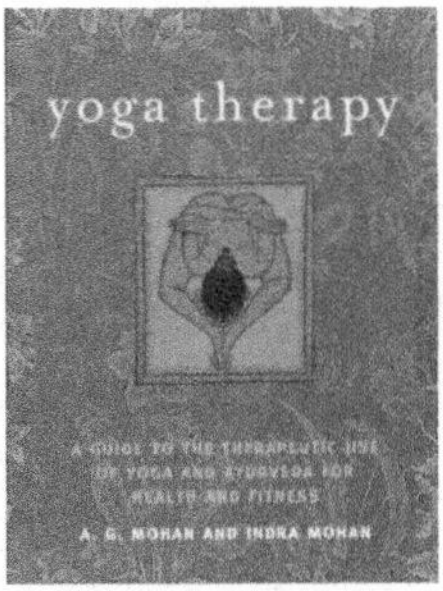

In the years that followed, Indra and I chose the name Svastha Yoga to represent an umbrella for his yoga teachings: the word *svastha* simply means health and wellbeing. That is the goal of yoga.

In 2004, our next book was published, titled *Yoga Therapy*, also dedicated to Krishnamacharya. The goal was to bring out the therapeutic aspects of his teachings.

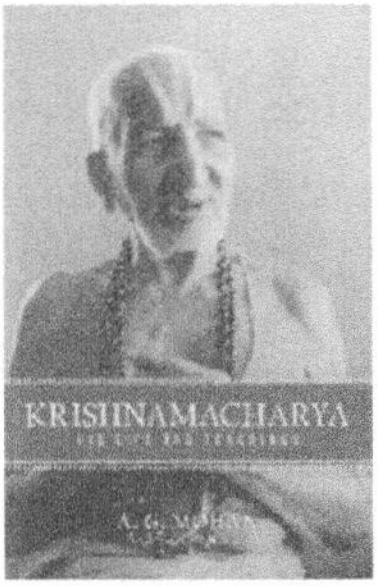

In 2010, with Ganesh, I wrote a book that is most dear to my heart, titled *Krishnamacharya: His Life and Teachings*. Starting with a biography of the master, I spoke about his greatness, chronicled my journey with him, and presented his teachings in a simple way, with numerous anecdotes.

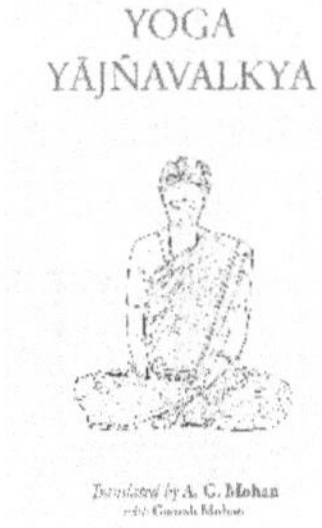

Turning our attention to traditional teachings, the *Yoga Yajnavalkaya* stood out. It was a traditional text that was held in high regard by Krishnamacharya, but not widely known. So, we translated and published that in 2013.

In 2015, we released a simple book on yoga, *Yoga Reminder*, following his ideal of making yoga accessible to every student.

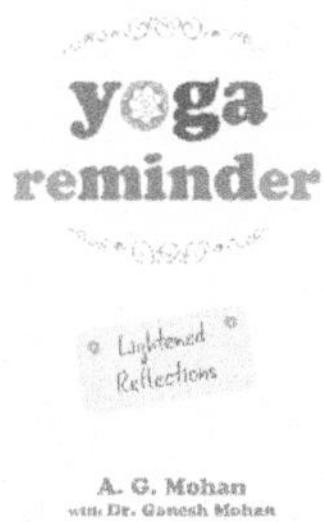

In 2017, we translated the Haṭha Yoga Pradīpikā with notes from Krishnamacharya. The master had so many unique insights on this classical haṭha yoga text that modern practitioners can benefit from.

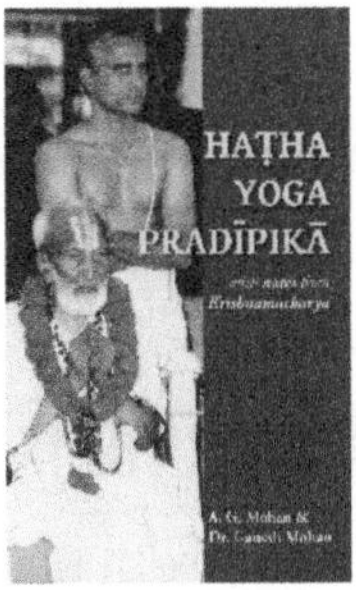

The book you are reading now is a continuation of these decades of effort in spreading his teachings.

Notes from classes

I wrote down everything that Krishnamacharya taught in my classes with him, practically verbatim. I accumulated several thousand pages of notes over 18 years. I have preserved all of it, from my first lessons to the last ones, spanning 1971 to 1989.

This book is a unique offering. It is literally one of a kind. Here, we present Krishnamacharya in his own words (translated into English, of course). This a special lens into his teachings and a window into traditional yoga studies.

We have selected portions from my notes that will be useful and comprehensible to a modern reader. Many of these teachings are not widely known.

Because of the years of personal classes with him, it is not surprising that I still sometimes dream of attending his classes. During my waking hours too, I have never been far from his teachings.

If I close my eyes, I can still see him sitting before me, speaking in his resonant voice, with his characteristic style and all the specific terms and language he preferred. So, we have followed not only his notes, but also his language and way of presentation.

This book is as direct a glimpse as any yoga reader can now receive of Krishnamacharya's teachings.

Studying with Krishnamacharya

A class with Krishnamacharya was never a prepared lecture. He did not make notes beforehand. He would speak from memory and the plan he had entirely in his mind. In some texts like the Haṭha Yoga Pradīpikā, where he did not see the necessity to memorize all the verses, he would occasionally refer to a printed version. In most other classes, he would have the text itself in memory.

In my case, as a long-term student, classes on some topics would continue for months. He would set the pace as he thought best. A sincere student does not go to a master like Krishnamacharya and decide on how they should learn. The teacher definitely knows better. While such an attitude can go wrong in the hands of lesser teachers, this was never a concern on my part, nor did the master's guidance ever fall short of what was best for me in all my years with him.

Nonetheless, Krishnamacharya was not a teacher who would go out of the way to instruct students. It was the student's responsibility to seek. It was only in my later years with him that he felt free enough with me to himself order me to do this or learn that. In the earlier years, he would ask me what I wanted to study—and, naturally, I would mostly always ask him to decide. Occasionally, I asked if he would teach me certain topics in greater detail, and he obliged. I learned pranayama in-depth and the esoteric aspects of the haṭha yoga by asking him to address those areas in my personal classes; this was several years into my association with him.

He would promptly dismiss any request or question that was not sincere, well-earned, and deeply considered. This meant that I would have to reflect on what he taught me, practice it if possible, and only then ask him a question about it. That said, he was always keen on ensuring that sound yoga should be taught. Therefore, he would answer questions related to how to pass on the teachings correctly.

How this book is structured

You might find the flow of this book very different from general books on yoga. That is intentional: the classes are written how Krishnamacharya said it. We wanted you to hear "his voice." Therefore, we have neither expanded nor summarized what he said. The goal of this book is to read like a series of dictated lectures directly from Krishnamacharya.

Of course, not all the points under a topic were always said together in a single lecture. Usually there would be much more material, as he would range across more topics. As a reader, you do not have years to sit through the lectures and work your way through all the points he said! Therefore, on some topics, we have chosen the points from multiple lectures and put them together. We have not modified those points; we have simply brought them together under a single heading.

To facilitate understanding, we have added footnotes and introductions to clarify Sanskrit words. We chose to add footnotes rather than intersperse the notes with the lecture—this helps to retain the feeling and flow of his thought better and connect you directly to him.

A few highlights

Krishnamacharya was never vague. He would not vacillate or present subjects with "maybe, could be, perhaps" attached. He was definitive. Such clarity and certainty were hallmarks of his teachings. One was never in any doubt as a student: I was in the presence of someone who had studied fully, in depth, and practiced what he was teaching.

When applying theory to students in practice, Krishnamacharya was always clear that practices should be taught according to the capacity of the student.

The master quoted extensively from so many traditional sources and texts (almost always from his memory). His astounding range of traditional studies meant that any class could link across many topics. You will find many such quotes and connections throughout the classes in this book—in reality, we had to limit them as a full presentation could be overwhelming to the modern reader.

May all be well

Krishnamacharya often used to end his lectures with the statement, "sarvaṃ śam." This means, "May everything, all living beings, be well."

With love and respect,

A. G. Mohan with Indra Mohan, Nitya Mohan & Ganesh Mohan

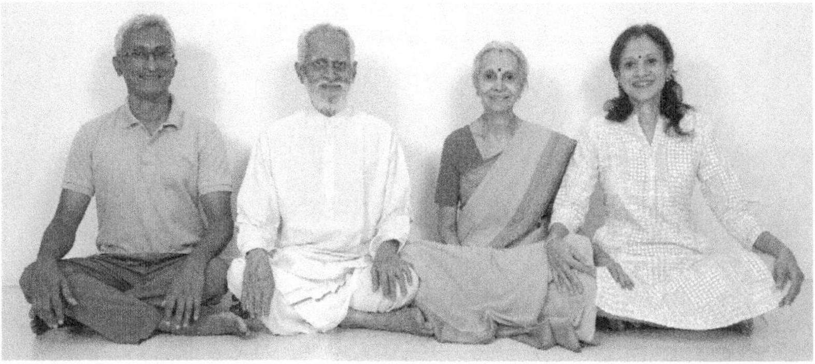

1 / The Yoga Path

In the 1970s, yoga was not widely known. There were only a few labels, unlike today. Krishnamacharya's presentation of the path of yoga only refers to the ancient texts and practices that existed in the centuries past. However, he was aware that the circumstances of life were changing in modern times. He himself lived through some of those changes.

There are many aspects of yoga that do not change, including the core presentations and practices. However, we need to modify many of these applications to make them possible for us today. Krishnamacharya was always sensitive to the importance of making practices possible for students. You will see that balance in his lectures in this section: ensuring that the key teachings do not change, but acknowledging and adapting to the circumstances that do inevitably change.

In his era, he had come across the radio. Towards his later years, he was aware of the small radio receivers that one could hold in hand and the advent of the television. He used to caution, "Be careful of the sounds and sights you put into your senses. They will distract the mind and upset its steadiness." Of course, such distractions were minimal then in comparison to what people face now with the internet!

On the other hand, he was also aware of technology being useful. He had recorded chanting and lectures for me to listen to and practice at home. This was possible only with a tape recorder. He was not fundamentally against technology; he was only keen that it should serve the progress of the student on the path of yoga toward health and peace.

We must be mindful of this balance: the world has changed a lot more in the forty years since these lectures, and will continue to shift further. We should not change certain values and practices because the human being has not changed. Yet, we should be willing to modify, adapt where relevant.

There is only one yoga and two merging yoga paths

Date: 1976 | Topic series: Yoga Sūtra

1. Nowadays, yoga has become more well-known. People speak of many types of yoga.
2. However, when we look at the traditional teachings, there are only two pathways. This is clear if you see Bhagavan Krishna's teachings in the Bhagavad Gita and Bhāgavata Purāṇa.
3. In the Bhagavad Gita, Krishna explains karma yoga to Arjuna. In the Bhagavata Purana, in Canto 11, Krishna explains jñāna yoga to Uddhava.[1]
4. Arjuna was not ready to practice jñāna yoga.[2] Therefore, Krishna did not advise him to leave everything and practice non-attachment (sanyāsa). This is why he does not also say anything about the siddhi-s. To Uddhava, however, he speaks about the siddhi-s.[3]

---

[1] Uddhava is a close friend and devotee of Krishna in the narration of his story in the epic, Bhāgavata Purāṇa. Krishna explains the intricacies of jñāna yoga to Uddhava in a section of the text called the Uddhava Gitā.

[2] Jñāna yoga requires the capacity of extended, deep meditation and is suitable for a person who is willing to let go of worldly activities and become a monk in the full-time pursuit of spiritual transformation.

[3] Special or extraordinary abilities may arise in the course of deep meditation practices, as the Yoga Sūtra says in Chapter 3. Therefore, a

5. In the Yoga Sūtra, in the first 22 sūtras (1.1-1.22), Patanjali explains the pathway of jñāna-yoga. This is yoga without Īśvara (Divine). It is sāṃkhya.

6. In Yoga Sūtra 1.23, he introduces Īśvara and tells us how to practice karma yoga with bhakti (devotion to Īśvara). This is why we can call yoga as sāṃkhya with Īśvara.

7. The pathway of the first 22 sūtra-s is possible only for a practitioner with a high degree of non-attachment (vairāgya). Only one in many millions of people may have such non-attachment nowadays. It is very rare.

8. Though these two pathways may seem different, they are the same. Bhagavan Krishna states this in the Bhagavad Gita (5.5), "The one who sees sāṃkhya and yoga as one, sees correctly."

9. Karma yoga with devotion to Īśvara (bhakti) is what Patanjali explains in Chapter 2 of the Yoga Sūtra. He starts with kriyā-yoga in Yoga Sūtra 2.1. These are not the kriyā-s of haṭha yoga. He means control over food, mantra meditation on one's personal deity, and the worship of that deity. This is kriyā-yoga here. If we continue to practice this pathway of kriyā-yoga, it will lead us to stillness of the mind (citta-nirodha).

The need for the right guru

Date: 1975, 1981, 1983 | Topic series: Yoga Sūtra, Mudrā, Vedic chanting

1. Yoga, singing, dancing, and Vedic chanting: these should be learned from a teacher.

---

practitioner following jñāna yoga must be aware of them. A person still on the path of karma yoga is not likely to encounter these siddhi-s yet, until their practice deepens further.

2. Among these, yoga is special because it brings us internal experiences and only through that do we have the realizations that lead to our progress. Vedic chanting should bring one-pointed focus of mind. For this, you need a right acharya.

3. The texts tell us that the teacher should first study yoga, then reflect, meditate, and practice it, and thereby realize it in direct experience.

4. In some of the ancient haṭha yoga texts, we can see excessive and unwarranted presentations. That is not sound. Only a good teacher can guide you wisely.

5. Only a good teacher who has comprehensive knowledge and practice will know what is possible and not possible, what is safe or dangerous, and what should be accepted and what should be discarded.

6. This becomes important when you read the haṭha yoga texts on topics like kriyā-s and pranayama. For example, there are recommendations to do pranayama with gāyatrī mantra and a 1:3:1 ratio.[4] This is not possible. We must understand the reading of the verse as "do it three times," meaning a ratio of 1:1:1.

7. There are many distortions of yoga practice that have been propagated over the years. In my younger days, I have debated against this and struggled to set this right. But times have changed. Only my own practice is affected by such efforts, so I have given up doing that.

8. The Haṭha Yoga Pradīpikā (1.65-66) says, "Success in yoga is not attained by merely studying the texts (śāstra-s). Success is not

---

[4] This means that the practitioner should repeat the 7-part gāyatrī mantra mentally once on inhalation, three times when holding after inhalation, and once on exhalation.

attained by wearing the clothes [of a yogi] or by talking about it." We must keep this in mind.

9. But know this for sure: As the Bhagavad Gita (2.40) says, if you understand the teaching of yoga correctly and practice it, even if only a little, you will definitely receive great benefits.

Prāṇa and mind: haṭha yoga and rāja yoga

Date: 1976 | Topic series: Yoga Sūtra, Haṭha Yoga Pradīpikā

1. A student asked me, "What is haṭha yoga? Is it different from rāja yoga?"[5]
2. In the ancient times, the Yoga Sūtra of Patanjali was known as rāja yoga. Nowadays, rāja yoga has become lectures!
3. In the same way, haṭha yoga has become āsana-s and kriyā-s.[6] Control over the mind cannot arise through just controlling the body.
4. In the Haṭha Yoga Pradīpikā (1.1), the commentator Bramhānanda says that the union of prāṇa and apāna is haṭha yoga. This means pranayama. He is referring to the fourth pranayama mentioned in the Yoga Sūtra of Patanjali (2.51).

---

[5] Generally, haṭha yoga refers to yoga focusing on physical practices, while rāja yoga refers to yoga focusing on meditative practices. Krishnamacharya explains what they are truly meant to be, and the deeper connections.

[6] Kriyā-s are bodily cleansing techniques such as nasal irrigation, inducing vomiting, swallowing a cloth and bringing it out, abdominal churning etc. They are presented in haṭha yoga texts such as the Haṭha Yoga Pradīpikā and Gheraṇḍa Samhitā.

5. From this, it is very clear that haṭha yoga is fundamentally pranayama.
6. Further, in the Haṭha Yoga Pradīpikā (2.76), Svātmārāma says, "Without haṭha yoga, rāja yoga cannot be achieved. And without rāja yoga, haṭha yoga is of no use. Therefore, both should be practiced until perfection is attained."
7. Here, what he means by haṭha yoga is stillness or control over the activity of prāṇa.[7] Rāja yoga is stillness or control over the activity of the mind.[8] There is no stillness of mind without control over prāṇa. Only if we practice both together can we achieve samādhi.
8. That is what the Haṭha Yoga Pradīpikā says in the next verse (2.77): "When holding the breath in pranayama, you must also focus the mind. Only then will you get the results of rāja yoga."
9. Also know this important point. Prāṇa is our power of activity. Mind is our power of will.[9] The two have a close connection.
10. Remember this pathway when you practice: both mind and prāṇa must be controlled together.
11. This is why, when starting the explanation of pranayama, the Haṭha Yoga Pradīpikā (2.1) says:

    athāsane dṛḍhe yogī vaśī hitamitāśanaḥ |
    gurūpadiṣṭamārgeṇa prāṇāyāmān samabhyaset ||1||

    "The yogi, having become competent in the practice of the āsana-s, with his senses under control, and following an

---

[7] "Haṭha yoga is prāṇa vṛtti nirodha."

[8] "Rāja yoga is citta vṛtti nirodha."

[9] "Prāṇa is kriyā śakti. Manas (mind) is icchā śakti."

appropriate and moderate diet, should practice prāṇāyāma, according to the instructions of his guru."

12. Here:

    a. The first point, *competence in asana*, means control over the body.

    b. The second point is to have control over the senses.

    c. The third point is to have control over food.

    d. The fourth point, *according to the instructions of the guru*, means to control the mind with the help of mantra.

    e. Along with all this, pranayama is to control the flow of the breath to make it long and subtle.

13. Do not practice in an uncontrolled or unsound way without accounting for all the above. It will lead to a bad name for yoga and for the one who teaches it.

Older and newer haṭha yoga in the classical texts

Date: 1975, 1976, 1981 | Topic series: Yoga Yājñavalkya, Yoga Sūtra, Haṭha Yoga Pradīpikā, Gheraṇḍa Samhitā

As I studied various classical haṭha yoga texts with Sri Krishnamacharya, he would compare them whenever relevant. Here I have collected the broad points of comparison he explained across lectures delivered in multiple years.

1. Among the classical haṭha yoga texts, the one that explains it in a way that is consistent with Vedic foundations is the Yoga Yājñavalkya.

2. The Haṭha Yoga Pradīpikā and Gheraṇḍa Samhitā are texts that came later. Some of the verses in these texts are copied from the Yoga Yājñavalkya.

3. These later texts also contain some inadvisable and unsafe practices. Much confusion has developed over centuries because of this.
4. A practitioner cannot succeed in yoga without the yama-s and niyama-s. The later texts do not give sufficient importance to the yama-s and niyama-s.
5. Only the Yoga Yājñavalkya explains the pathway of yoga systematically. It details a proper, stepwise approach (krama), following the eight limbs of yoga.
6. The Yoga Yājñavalkya gives us a detailed description of prāṇa and the nāḍī-s before embarking on the process of purifying them.
7. It is also the view of Yājñavalkya that the impurities in the body can be purified by control over food, and the practice of pranayama and mantra. Hence, the physical cleansing techniques of the kriyā-s are not mentioned in his text.
8. In later texts such as the Haṭha Yoga Pradīpikā, it is recommended that the physical cleansing of the kriyā-s should be done before pranayama. But even they mention that sages such as Yājñavalkya do not consider these kriyā-s to be necessary (Haṭha Yoga Pradīpikā 2.36). This tells us that the Yoga Yājñavalkya is the older text.
9. The Gheraṇḍa Samhitā is of the opinion that body should be cleansed by the kriyā-s as the first step in haṭha yoga. Therefore, it mentions these before even asana.
10. The Yoga Yājñavalkya does not explain the bandha-s and mudrā-s like the other texts. It talks only about ṣaṇmukhī-mudrā for the practice of meditation.

Chapters in the Haṭha Yoga Pradīpikā	Chapters in the Gheraṇḍa Samhitā	Chapters in the Yoga Yājñavalkya
1. Asanas 2. Pranayama & Kriyās 3. Mudrās & Bandhas 4. Nādānusandhāna	1. Kriyā-s 2. Asana 3. Mudrā 4. Pratyāhāra 5. Pranayama 6. Dhyana 7. Samādhi	1. Yama 2. Niyama 3. Asanas 4. Prāṇa & Nāḍī-s 5. Nāḍīśodhana pranayama 6. Pranayama-s 7. Pratyāhāra 8. Dhāraṇā 9. Dhyāna 10. Samādhi 11. Samādhi & Yoga karma 12. Summary

Light on haṭha yoga: introducing the Haṭha Yoga Pradīpikā

Date: 1976 | Topic series: Haṭha Yoga Pradīpikā

This was the first lecture in the series on the Hatha Yoga Pradīpikā, on 17 July 1976. Krishnamacharya would start with an auspicious verse. In his preference, this was to his Vaishnavite acharya. Then he would ask me to chant the verses with him. We would chant the verses we had covered recently, and then take up from where we had left off in the last session.

These classes took place once a week. So, I requested him to record the Haṭha Yoga Pradīpikā chanting on tape so that I could listen to them at home and familiarize myself with the verses. He consented and we recorded the chanting.

1. Ha is the prāṇa (life force) that flows in the sūrya nāḍī (channel of the sun) known as piṅgalā. This channel is connected with the right nostril. The Bīja Nighaṇṭu has given the name “ha” to this vāyu.[10]

2. The vāyu (life force) that flows in the left nostril is designated by the sound ṭha.

3. When the ha and ṭha vāyu-s that flow in these two nāḍī-s (channels) join in the central suṣumnā,[11] that is called haṭha yoga. This book shows us the easy pathway to achieve this.

4. The word pradīpa means a shining lamp. This book is the lamp that illuminates haṭha yoga.

5. There is no yoga text that does not start with a prayer.

6. Haṭha yoga is a ladder. The higher steps of this ladder are rāja yoga.

7. This text mentions two lineages: the muni-s such as Vasiṣṭa and yogi-s such as Matsyendra. Vasiṣṭa is one of the seven great traditional sages.[12] Muni means one who is silent. What this

---

[10] We can take “vāyu” to be approximately synonymous with “prāṇa” in this context.

[11] Suṣumnā is the channel in the center of the spine to the crown of the head.

[12] They are known as the sapta ṛṣi-s or literally, seven sages. The list of names varies according to the traditional source.

means is that, when a muni is asked a question, he is able to show the practice and be an example, and not just speak about the topic.

8. Matsyendranātha is from the Natha tradition of yogis. Kuraṇṭa is one of the yogis in that tradition. This text explains the asanas given and approved by the sages such as Vasiṣṭa and yogis such as Matsyendranātha.

9. How many asanas are there? Dhyānabindu Upaniṣad says, "There are as many asanas as there are types of living beings."

10. This text also explains pranayama. Without prāṇa, there is no life. The text says, "As long as there is prāṇa in the body, there is life." (Haṭha Yoga Pradīpikā 2.3)

11. Asana is for maintaining the strength and fitness of the body. But it is pranayama that bestows long life.

12. The text begins with Śrī Ādinātha. Śrī denotes the goddess Lakṣmī and auspiciousness. Ādinātha is lord Śiva. You can consider that this means lord Viṣnu also. As the famous poet Kālidāsa prays to lord Śiva and Pārvati, but his verse can be interpreted as praying to lord Viṣnu and Lakṣmī also, we can adopt the same principle here.[13]

13. Ha denoting piṅgalā, the channel of the sun, refers to prāṇa. Ṭha denoting iḍā, the channel of the moon, refers to apāna.

---

[13] This is a reference to the opening prayer verse of the famous work Raghuvamśa. The Sanskrit wording of whom he is offering salutations to can be interpreted in two ways, by splitting it differently. Split one way (pārvatī + parameśvarau) it refers to goddess Pārvatī and lord Śiva. Split another way (pārvatīpa + rameśvarau) it refers to lord Śiva and lord Viṣṇu, with their respective goddesses.

14. Therefore, the union of prāṇa and apāna is pranayama. Here the pranayama referred to is the fourth pranayama mentioned in the Yoga Sūtra (2.51).

15. In practice, the Bhagavad Gita (4.29) says that the prāṇa and apāna should be united. There is no difference of opinion between the major traditional teachers (ācārya-s) on this topic. Here, apāna means exhalation and prāṇa means inhalation.

16. Kevala kumbhaka, the fourth pranayama in the Yoga Sūtra (2.51), can be attained through haṭha yoga. This is the pathway of Gorakṣanātha. This is also the pathway to rāja yoga.

17. Rāja means king. Uniting with the king is rāja yoga. Here, the king is the Divine (paramātma), as the Vedic mantras say in Maha Nārāyaṇa Upaniṣad.[14]

18. Another meaning is that rāja yoga is the highest, greatest among different yoga-s. Rāja-sthāna means the head of the body, the place of the sahasrāra (the crown of the head). The seed mantra to attain that is OM. Haṭha yoga is therefore essential for rāja yoga, because only if prāṇa enters the suṣumnā channel, it can reach the top of the head.

Eight limbs of yoga and what we can practice now (yama, niyama, asana)

Date: 1975 | Topic series: Yoga Today

Sri Krishnamacharya delivered a series of lectures under the title "Yoga Today." He addressed the theme, "In the times of today, what yoga is possible or not, what can we practice?"

---

[14] The mantra refers to the Divine as rājā or king.

1. I will first speak about the eight limbs of yoga.[15] Then we will be able to analyze and understand what is possible and what is not in the existing conditions in the kali yuga[16] now.

2. In the Yoga Sūtra, Patanjali gives us five yama-s.[17] Among these, non-harmfulness (ahimsā) cannot be fully followed by us now in the manner explained in the sūtra-s. We can only do it to some extent.

3. Speaking the truth, avoiding untruth (satya) and non-stealing (asteya)—these are also not possible in the way explained in the sūtra-s.

   Stealing wealth, corruption, has increased. So has stealing the good works of others or avoiding doing good actions because of laziness. Therefore, it is difficult to follow truthfulness and non-stealing in the ancient ways.[18]

---

[15] The eight limbs of yoga are yama, niyama, āsana, prāṇāyāma, pratyāhara, dhāranā dhyāna, and samādhi.

[16] The four yuga-s are the cosmological time scales in ancient Vedic presentation: kṛta yuga, tretā yuga, dvāpara yuga, and kali yuga. We are now in the last, the kali yuga. Spiritual decline is supposed to happen from the first to the last, hence people now are less capable of doing yoga practices than the earlier times.

[17] Yama-s, first of the eight limbs of yoga, are restraints of thought, speech, and behavior. They are five: ahimsā (non-harmfulness), satya (not lying), asteya (not stealing), bramhacarya (control over sex), aparigraha (non-acquisitiveness).

[18] Steya = stealing. Stealing wealth: dhana-steya; dhana = wealth. Stealing the good actions of others: dharma-steya; dharma = ethical conduct.

4. Control over sexual behavior (bramhacarya) is possible because it is in each person's hands to follow. It does not depend on another person.

5. Non-acquisitiveness (aparigraha): this is doable with difficulty. As Manu said, "Even if you can take more, limit yourself to what you need." Nowadays, that limit is crossed. People are lost in desire.

6. Under the niyamas,[19] outer cleanliness and inner purity (śauca) and contentment, satisfaction (santoṣa), can be practiced to some extent.

7. Tapas is derived from the Sanskrit root word "to heat." The body, made of the five bhūta-s,[20] is heated by tapas. The body is like a vessel that principally contains water. We can purify it by heat with fire (agni). By practicing tapas, we can keep the body well. Only through tapas, one can master the senses. The most important practice for tapas is moderation in food habits. Do not overeat.

8. Svādhyāya is Vedic chanting. The continuity of these traditions has been interrupted now. So, at least, buy and read a translation of the Vedas to the extent you can.

---

[19] Niyama-s, second of the eight limbs of yoga, are five observances, practices to quiet activity: śauca (cleanliness), santoṣa (contentment), tapas (tolerating discomfort), svādhyāya (mantra meditation and studying the traditional texts), īśvara-praṇidhāna (letting go of results of actions, connection to the Divine).

[20] The five bhūta-s are space, air, fire, water, earth. They do not literally mean these elements. They refer to the various qualities of physical reality represented in summary by these five.

9. Īśvara praṇidhāna: First, cultivate good company for ten months. There were two parrots. One of the two parrots was brought up in a peaceful household. The other was brought up in a butcher's house. The former would speak good words, the latter would speak harsh words. So, for faith in the Divine to grow, we must keep good company.[21]

10. Asana is position of the body. It is to be stable, without shaking. You should not have any pain or discomfort. Dhyanabindu Upaniṣad Chapter 23 says that there are as many asanas as there are types of living beings in the world.

11. Asanas should be done according to the state of the person's body. Asanas can be divided into two types. Lean persons should do bṛmhaṇa practice. Fat persons should do langhana practice.[22] That means: Lean persons can do retention of breath after inhale. Fat persons can do retention of breath after exhale.

12. Normally, our breath is at a rate of 12-15 per minute. We should reduce that. So, take deep, long breaths.

13. Everyone does not need to do all asanas. Nor do all asanas need to be done at all times.

14. The benefit of doing asanas is good health. Expulsion of wastes from the body will proceed normally. Heat and cold in the body will be in balance.

---

[21] A ten-month time is called a samvatsara in Sanskrit, a traditional duration for certain practices.

[22] These two Sanskrit words are drawn from ayurveda. Bṛmhaṇa therapies are those that increase body mass. Langhana therapies are those that decrease body mass. Krishnamacharya used to say, "lean person" and "fat person."

15. If you do paścimatanāsana (seated forward bend), you must follow it with pūrvatanāsana (seated backward bend). This is called pratikriyāsana (counter-pose).[23]

16. We may suffer from many diseases. Therefore, many asanas are described to help remove them.

Eight limbs of yoga and what we can practice now (pranayama)

Date: 1975 | Topic series: Yoga Today

1. Pranayama should be done after asana. Through asana the actions of our body are purified. The Shārīra Upaniṣad mentions this.

2. In south India, Vedic rituals are practiced for purification. In north India, for purification, mantra and devotional practices are used more.

3. If we do pranayama properly, the result is that clouding of our consciousness diminishes.

4. Prāṇa is not air. Vyāsa explains this in the Bramha Sūtra, Chapter 3.

5. We must lengthen the prāṇa. That is the meaning of the word āyāma.

[23] Literally, prati = opposite, kriyā = action, āsana = posture.

6. The prāṇa consists of ten vāyu-s.[24] If we use these ten vāyu-s properly, our five instruments of actions and five senses of perception will function well.[25]

7. Remember this: to receive these benefits, we must practice pranayama with concentration.

8. The primary place of the prāṇa is the center of the chest, the heart region (hṛdaya).

9. There are four circles in the heart center.[26]

10. We must practice pranayama every day for a long life and good health. Prāṇa should always be guarded carefully.

11. Pranayama may be done with mantra and without mantra.[27]

12. Pranayama can also be classified as being done with equal ratio of inhalation and exhalation (sama-vṝtti) or unequal ratios of inhalation and exhalation (viṣama-vṛtti).

13. Pranayama with equal ratio is mentioned in the Bhagavad Gita (5.27) which says, "Make the inhale and exhale flowing in the nostrils equal..."

---

[24] Vāyu means "air" and here it refers to categories of the functions of prāṇa. These functions are divided into ten in yoga texts such as the Yoga Yājñavalkya.

[25] Five instruments of action are two arms, two legs, and the tongue. Five senses of perception are sound, touch, sight, taste, and smell.

[26] The four circles are the Divine, individual consciousness, prāṇa, and the mind.

[27] With a mantra = sa-mantraka. Without a mantra = a-mantraka.

14. Pranayama with unequal ratios is also mentioned in the Bhagavad Gita (4.30): "Let the inhale be offered to the exhale and the exhale be offered to inhale..."

15. After inhale, hold, and press the pelvic floor down. Join prāṇa with apāna. After exhale, keep the pelvic floor lifted. Join apāna with prāṇa.

16. Mantra should be done along with pranayama. Mantra can be one or two syllables, up to eight syllables.

17. Pranayama leads to good memory. It should be done with sāttvic food and control over the urge for sex.

18. Normal pulse rate of a person may be 72. It can be reduced to 45 with good pranayama. It could even be brought down further.

19. Gaze at the tip of the nose while doing pranayama.

20. Pranayama practice should give us both visible results and hidden results.

21. What pranayamas can be practiced in the present day? Ujjāyī, śītalī, śītkārī, and naḍīśodhana.

22. Pranayama practice can lead to the state of no exhale, no inhale.[28]

23. Dharma is that which supports you, prevents you from falling (from the path of ethics and yoga). Do pranayama while adhering to dharma (yama-s and niyama-s).

---

[28] This is termed kevala-kumbhaka: only suspension, no movement of the breath.

2 / Asana & Mudrā

I started studying asanas with Krishnamacharya in 1973. Initially, he taught me long, deep, smooth breathing along with movement. He did not introduce the important bhavana-s in asana then. Of course, he was right to limit what he taught me—as a beginner student, I would not have been able to understand and apply those deeper practices right away.

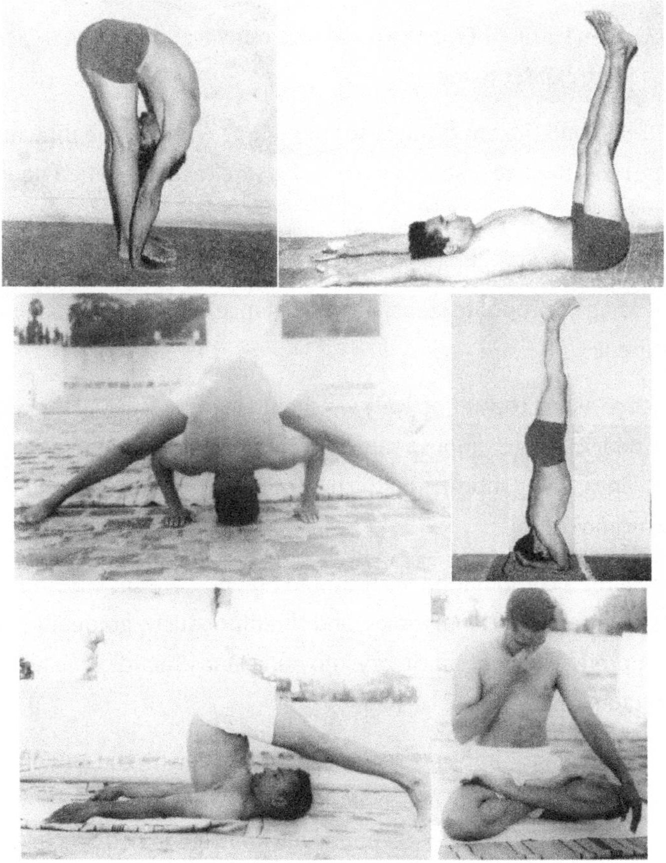

A. G. Mohan in 1973

Instead, when I asked to study theory and philosophy with him, he began teaching me the Praśna Upaniṣad because it would complement my asana and pranayama practice. In those classes, he explained the prāṇa bhavana-s and much more.

In 1975, when he taught me the Yoga Yājñavalkya, he explained how agni and prāṇa are crucial to health and yoga practice.

In 1975-76, during lectures on the Yoga Sūtra he described the three agni-s in the body and how we can relate to them, physically and spiritually.

In 1977, when he taught me the ritual of sandhyāvandana, the topic of agni became clearer to me.

In 1986-87, I had the opportunity to spend time with him clearing my doubts. I was then also able to look back at the teachings I had deepened over years.

Along the way, he taught me many principles of effectively applying asana: using appropriate steps, finding balance, suiting the teachings to the student.

To practice asana truly effectively we should learn at least all the above: the art and science of appropriate application to the student (anga, krama, vinyasa and more), and the inner connections (prāṇa, agni, bhavana and more).

This requires a combination of study and practice. We should study and reflect on these traditional topics, and simultaneously, gradually bring our comprehension of that theory into our asana practice. One will support the other.

This pathway takes time and personal dedication, with the guidance of a sound teacher, ultimately not too different from the way Krishnamacharya gradually deepened my knowledge and practice as I studied with him.

In his lectures, Krishnamacharya would sometimes mention his life experiences in his earlier years. He would refer to people he had met, taught, or treated—to give examples and help me understand better.

Though Krishnamacharya was originally from south India, he spent a lot of time in north India in his earlier years. One phase of his travels was during his studies, where he spent time in the traditional universities and elsewhere during his breaks. The second phase of his exposure was after the completion of his studies. He said that he had moved around for a while, gaining exposure to various practices and applications of traditional studies, somewhat like a wandering monk.

He used to say that the practices of kriyā-s and mudrā-s was more prevalent in the northern regions of India rather than the south. This was because of the bairāgi-s, wandering monks, being in greater number there. They had to eat what was given and put up with varying climates in different places. This was one of the reasons, he felt, the kriyā-s had more use there. If one is settled in a place with a daily routine of food and environment, the kriyā-s become less relevant. A more limited set of practices is sufficient—safer and as effective. The results of some of the kriyā-s can be attained through asana, pranayama, and diet changes.

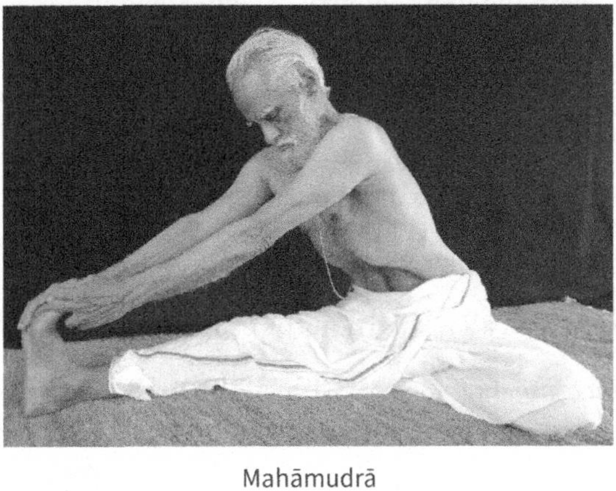

Mahāmudrā

Therefore, when studying the Haṭha Yoga Pradīpikā first, and then the Gheraṇḍa Samhitā in 1980-81, he gave directions on which practices to avoid, substitutions for some practices, and how to modify some other practices.

When teaching me chapter 3 of the Haṭha Yoga Pradīpikā, he stopped and said, "The further materials are not necessary. My guru has told me not to teach these. It is enough if you learn viparīta karaṇī mudrā from me." In Krishnamacharya's view, viparīta karaṇī mudrā, mahāmudrā, taḍāga mudrā, and ṣanmukhī mudrā were most important and sufficient. Apart from this, the aṅjali mudrā especially in asana, āvahana mudrā in sandhyāvandana, as well as mṛgi mudrā in pranayama, were recommended by him.

Yoga-vidyā: the knowledge of yoga

Krishnamacharya's definition of learning yoga

samanaska sa-vinyāsa sa-pratikriyā yukta sagarbha agarbha bhedamukha yamaniyamādi samādhi yukta yoga vidyā |

samanaska: with sattva and mindfulness

sa-vinyāsa: with the methodology of right steps

sa-pratikriyā: with balance

yukta: along with

sagarbha (samantraka): with mantra

agarbha (amantraka): or without mantra

bhedamukha: with all its divisions or branches

yamaniyamādi samādhi yukta: with all the limbs from the yama-s and niyama-s to samādhi *yoga vidyā*: such is the knowledge of yoga (to be learnt from a proper guru)

Importance of vinyāsa

vinā vinyāsa yogena āsanādīn na kārayet |

Do not do asana and other practices without the proper application of structured goals and steps (vinyasa) and without yoga (mindfulness and stillness of mind).

udāttādi svarairhīnaḥ yathā vedo nirarthakaḥ |

aṅganyāsādibhirhīnaḥ yathā mantro nirarthakaḥ ||

prāṇāyāmaḥ kālagaṇānāṁ apāhāya nirarthakaḥ |

tathā vinyāsa hīnañca yogāsanaṁ anarthakam ||

Just as recitation of the Vedas done without proper notes will not yield the proper results...

Just as mantra done without appropriate ritual will not yield the desired result...

Just as pranayama done without structure will not yield the desired result...

Similarly, asanas done without proper vinyāsa (structured goals and steps) will not yield desired result (may be harmful).

Prāṇa bhāvana-s in asana and pranayama

Date: 1973, 1975 | Topic series: Praśna Upaniṣad, Yoga Yājñavalkya

These bhāvana-s are important when we practice asana and pranayama. They are essential for health as well as spiritual transformation.

1. *Prāṇa sancāra bhāvana:*[29] When we breathe in and out during asana and pranayama, we must feel the prāṇa expanding from our heart center, its origin, and filling our body on inhalation, and feel the prāṇa returning to our heart center on exhalation.
2. This prāṇa sancāra bhāvana is important to help the assimilation of the food we eat into all our body tissues.
3. *Prāṇa agni bhāvana:*[30] When we inhale, the prāṇa is flowing down and in toward the agni in the abdomen. This increases the agni. When we exhale, the place of apāna in the lower abdomen moves up toward the agni in the abdomen. This burns the impurities in the body. On exhale, prāṇa then removes these impurities from the body.
4. This prāṇa agni bhāvana is not only about removing the impurities of the body, but also from the mind.
5. *Prāṇa kartā bhāvana*: This bhāvana is important for spiritual transformation. The origin of the prāṇa in the body is the heart center, which is also the place of the Divine and our consciousness. When you breathe, do it with the feeling that the doer is the Divine in the form of prāṇa. This will diminish ego and attachment.
6. The Taittiriya Upaniṣad says: Prāṇa is the head because it is the most important, it is the doer. To manage this, we should practice prāṇa kartā bhāvana. Vyāṇa is the right hand, it is everywhere in the body and is responsible for movement. To manage this, we should practice prāṇa sancāra bhāvana. Apāna is the left hand, it is the remover of impurities. To manage this, we should practice prāṇa agni bhāvana. The space between the prāṇa and apāna is the center. This is the space of samāna vāyu.

---

[29] Sancāra here means *to flow*.

[30] Agni means *fire*. Here it refers principally to the digestive fire in the abdomen.

The ground is udāna vāyu which anchors our life force in the body.

Three agni-s for wellbeing: first in the abdomen

Date: 1975 | Topic series: Yoga Sūtra

1. There are three agni-s in our body. If we keep them in good function, we will not have ill-health in body and mind. I will explain their name, location, and practices.
2. The three agni-s are important for fitness, yoga therapy, and spiritual transformation,[31] including the siddhi-s.
3. The first is called jāṭharāgni. It is located in the abdomen.[32]
4. To keep this agni in good function, use taḍāga-mudrā with good breathing.
5. Another name given to this agni is vaiśvānara-agni, in the Bhagavad Gita (15.14). The implication of this word is that all living beings have it.[33] Bhagavan Krishna says that he, as the Divine, is this agni in all beings, and supports the digestion of food by working along with prāṇa.
6. We can also meditate on this vaiśvānara-agni, that supports all digestion, as a representation of the Divine.

---

[31] He refers to śikṣā-krama, cikitsā-krama, and ādhyātmika krama-s here.

[32] The word *jaṭhara* means "abdomen." Krishnamacharya would occasionally mention the English word "stomach," referring to entire abdominal region.

[33] *Viśva* means universal and *nara* refers to all living beings.

7. In haṭha yoga, the place of this abdominal agni is referred to as the maṇipūra cakra.
8. In the Yoga Sūtra (3.29), this place is called the navel cakra (nābhi cakra). By meditating on the place of this cakra, we gain insight into the configuration of the body.
9. This abdominal agni is vital to our well-being. It is a center of activity and has more of the quality of rajas among the three guṇa-s (sattva, rajas, and tamas).
10. Agni and prāṇa together purify all the nāḍī-s. But that function depends on the posture, breath, and bhāvana we use.

Three agni-s for wellbeing: second in the crown of the head

Date: 1975 | Topic series: Yoga Sūtra

1. This is called the *jñāna-agni,* the fire of knowledge of discernment.
2. The place of this agni is the crown of the head.
3. This agni supports the function of clarity and discernment in our mind.
4. The Bhagavad Gita (4.19) refers to this agni: all karma (impulse to action) is destroyed in the power of this fire, jñāna-agni.
5. The Yoga Sūtra (4.29) refers to this agni too.[34] It destroys the impulses of the kleśa-s by burning them.

---

[34] The Yoga Sūtra uses the term prasaṅkhyāna agni.

6. In our normal lives, this agni helps us with worldly and beneficial discernment: what we should do or not do, and what will lead us to happiness or unhappiness.
7. The postures related to this agni are headstand and shoulderstand. This is also connected to the practice referred to in the Yoga Sūtra 3.32.[35]
8. Being a center of discernment and clarity, it has more of the quality of sattva among the three guṇa-s (sattva, rajas, tamas).
9. The connections to the functions of the mind are greater with this agni. The connections to the function of the body are greater with the abdominal agni (jāṭharāgni).
10. In haṭha yoga, we say that if we cleanse the nāḍi-s through the practices of asana and pranayama, we will be able to experience the cakra-s in the body. The Vedic pathway is that we can achieve the same results by using agni, prāṇa, and mantra. This is described in the Yoga Yājñavalkya.
11. To keep the abdominal agni healthy, our food must be appropriate. To keep the agni at the crown of the head well, we must follow the yama-s and niyamas and manage our mind appropriately.
12. Jñāna, knowledge, can be divided into two categories. The first category is knowledge related to worldly matters. This knowledge is connected with the ājñā cakra (at the center of the eyebrows). The second category is knowledge related to one's self, spiritual knowledge. This knowledge is connected with the sahasrāra cakra (at the crown of the head).

---

[35] See the chapter *Mind & Meditation*, section *Light in the crown cakra, headstand practice, siddha-s.*

Three agni-s for wellbeing: third in the heart center

Date: 1975 | Topic series: Yoga Sūtra

1. This is called the *dahara-agni.*[36]
2. The place of this agni is the heart center.
3. It is realized through meditation.
4. Useful postures are padmasana (lotus) and related seated postures.
5. The Bhagavad Gita (10.20, 18.61) explains that the Divine is present in the heart center, in the region of this agni.
6. The Nārāyaṇa Upaniṣad speaks about this expansively.
7. In haṭha yoga, the place of this dahara agni is referred to as the anāhata cakra (heart cakra).
8. In the Yoga Sūtra, Vyāsa's commentary refers to this place as the "heart lotus" in 3.1. By practicing prolonged absorptive meditation on this region, the yogi experiences the nature of consciousness (3.35).
9. This agni in the heart center is the support for the other two agni-s in the abdomen and crown of the head. It is the source of illumination.
10. The abdominal agni is closely connected with food. The agni in the crown is closely related to the mind. The agni in the heart center is closely related to prāṇa and consciousness.

---

[36] *Dahara* refers to the place, the subtle inner space, of the heart.

11. This is why the Upaniṣads speak of the flowering of the heart lotus and the Yoga Yājñavalkya refers to pranayama as the practice to help with that.

Yoga Sūtra on asana: stable and comfortable

Date: 1976 | Topic series: Yoga Sūtra

1. Vyāsa says, "So far, we have explained the yama-s and niyama-s, with the signs of their success. Now we will explain asana."
2. What is asana? It is to be sthira—stable, without shaking. And to be sukha—comfortable.
3. Why do we need this stability? As you have learned in the Vedas in the Aruṇa Praṣna of the Taittirīya Āraṇyaka,[37] we chant, "May we be blessed with a stable (strong) body." It is necessary for health.
4. Patanjali has included sukha (comfortable) here because asana should not cause danger. It should be pleasant.
5. Vyāsa says, we should do asana with support or assistance.[38] All asanas can be done with or without support. For instance, shoulderstand can be done in a supported version and an unsupported version.
6. If someone cannot do the unsupported version, we can begin with the supported version. For example, if someone is unable to stay upright for pranayama, we can give him a support for the spine.

---

[37] This is the first section of the Taittirīya Āraṇyaka.

[38] Vyāsa's commentary uses with the word "sopāśraya" which separates into "sahita upāśraya" meaning "with support."

7. By practicing the unsupported versions of asanas, the lightness of our body increases.

8. Vyāsa says, "asana such as these." No number is specified because asanas are countless. Dhyanabindu Upaniṣad says that there are as many asanas as there are types of living beings.

9. When you start practicing asanas, you may not have stability in the body at first. There will be some effort, and so you may face some discomfort too. But if you continue to practice, you will gradually find both stability and comfort. As the Bhagavad Gita (18.37) says, this is sāttvic pleasure—it is initially difficult but becomes pleasant later.

10. Like a candy that is soaking in sugar syrup, the experience becomes sweet all the way through, gradually. For this to happen, we must continue with sound asana practice.

Three divisions in the pathway of asana practice

Date: 1976 | Topic series: Yoga Sūtra

1. Asana has three limbs (aṅga-s) termed śikṣā-aṅga, cikitsā-aṅga, and upāsana-aṅga.

2. The first, śikṣā-aṅga, is teaching asanas in an appropriate order (krama) to a person who is healthy.

3. The second, cikitsā-aṅga, is teaching asanas in an appropriate order to a person who is suffering from ill-health (disease).

4. The third, upāsana-aṅga, is spiritual. It is dhāraṇā, dhyāna, samādhi (pathway of meditation).

5. All these three should be practiced together, just as all the eight limbs of the yoga of Patanjali are practiced together. This is because we cannot separate the body and mind.

6. Bhagavan Patanjali has not mentioned bhakti-aṅga (the path of devotion) separately. This is because, in his view, through the pathway of meditation, bhakti will develop automatically.
7. If we grow a banana tree, our main goal is the banana fruit. However, we also get the other products like the stem, flower, and leaf.[39] Similarly, bhakti will also arise as a natural result of the meditation practice.
8. Śikṣā-aṅga can be divided into two:
    a. Training the student.
    b. Training of teachers.
9. Cikitsā-aṅga can be divided into two:
    a. Treating minor diseases.
    b. Treating major diseases
10. Upāsana-aṅga can be divided into two:
    a. For material benefits and siddhi-s.
    b. For freedom (mokṣa).

Teaching a healthy individual (śikṣā-aṅga)

Date: 1976 | Topic series: Yoga Sūtra

1. There are various krama-s (orders or ways of teaching).
2. We should know how to teach each asana individually.
3. We should know how to group asanas in teaching.

---

[39] The various parts of the banana tree are all useful. The banana stem and flowers can be cooked and eaten. The leaf can be used as a plate.

4. Both of these have an initial phase, main phase, and the after-phase.

5. All rituals such as sandhyāvandana and even weddings have these three phases. The asana practice also has these phases—the teacher must know them.

6. In the traditional Vedic wedding ceremony, for instance, the main phase has the key action: the couple clasp their hands together in a sign of their union and seal their vow with seven symbolic steps together with mantras.

7. In yoga, the main phase is meditation with mantra. We do asana and pranayama as the initial phase to prepare for this.

8. Traditionally, when learning Vedic chanting, the student has an initial phase of learning the chanting by repetition. Then after proficiency, a period of time is set aside to revise the chants he has learned. This cycle repeats in every year of learning. Similarly, every year, you must set aside time to revise all the practices that you have learned. This includes all the three aṅga-s (śikṣā-aṅga, cikitsā-aṅga, upāsana-aṅga) in self-application.

Asana requires breath and mind to work with the body

Date: 1976 | Topic series: Yoga Sūtra

This is an explanation of Yoga Sūtra 2.47.

1. How can the body be stable and comfortable in asana?

2. Mastery in asana cannot be achieved just by controlling the body. Only with control over the breath and mind will asana be mastered.

3. Patanjali uses the word *effort* (prayatna) in the Yoga Sūtra. He means the effort of life, which is the breath. We need to make this loose, break it.[40] That is, we need to practice long inhale and exhale.

4. The Yoga Sūtra describes two types of results for every practice—the temporary or material benefit, and the permanent benefit leading to mokṣa. If we want permanent benefit, we need to include meditation.

5. For this, Patanjali includes the phrase ananta-samāpatti which refers to meditation on Ādi-śeṣa.[41]

6. Alternatively, because Patanjali is considered to be an incarnation of Ādi-śeṣa, we can meditate on Patanjali himself.

7. A third way of understanding this is: Ādi-śeṣa can refer to our own prāṇa or life force. Ādi means "in the beginning." Śeṣa means "what is left over." Along with our consciousness, what is hidden or subtle (what it comes along with) is prāṇa. It is there from the moment of conception, all the time with the fetus. When the fetus is born, the five prāṇa-s are inside the baby, and because of that it draws in the air from outside, by breathing.

---

[40] The Yoga Sūtra 2.47 uses the words prayatna meaning "special effort" and śaithilya meaning "looseness, breaking up."

[41] Literally, the word ananta means "endless." Traditionally, the word ananta can refer to the divine serpent, known as Ādi-śeṣa, upon whom the Divine in the form of the deity Viṣṇu sleeps. Ādi-śeṣa embodies the quality of stability as he supports the origin of the entire universe. He also simultaneously embodies the quality of comfort, as he remains soft enough to be a bed for Viṣṇu. Sri Krishnamacharya offers an additional interpretation of the verse here, making it practical in our body too.

8. Therefore, ananta ("the endless") or Ādi-śeṣa ("what is hidden from the beginning") also refers to our own prāṇa. Patanjali is also saying that we can meditate on our own prāṇa. This is done through prāṇa-kartā-bhāvana (experiencing prāṇa as the doer).[42]

9. A student who does not practice with such bhāvana, is doing asana like animals do. They also assume such postures.

10. When you do bhāvana, the mind becomes stable. It is not disturbed. Because the senses do not move outwards, there is a feeling of pleasantness. Therefore, you *must* do bhāvana in asana with long inhale and exhale.

11. However, in cikitsā-aṅga (yoga as therapy), if the student cannot do long inhale and exhale, they can just breathe as long as possible for them, and combine it with such bhāvana.

12. A yoga teacher must have control over the senses. However, many yoga teachers are doing just asana now.

13. Your skin complexion will improve if you do asana properly. You will see this in time.

Mudrā-s in the yoga texts

Date: 1980 | Topic series: Gheraṇḍa Samhitā

1. A mudrā is a seal. Nowadays, you will see that when government officials need to examine something, they "seal" it.

2. In the context of yoga, the purpose of this seal is to examine and cleanse the 24 tattva-s of prakṛti. The goal is to realize oneself as

---

[42] See the chapter *Asana & Mudra*, section *Prāṇa bhāvana s in asana and pranayama*.

consciousness through this process. We examine and cleanse the activities of the mind, senses, and the flow of the breath.

3. The yoga path of Patanjali, includes five mudrā-s to cleanse five aspects of oneself (25 tattva-s of Sāṃkhya divided into five groups).

4. The Gheraṇḍa Samhitā has 25 mudrā-s to cleanse the prakṛti. This includes mudrā-s to cleanse the five bhūta-s (space, air, fire, water, earth). The Haṭha Yoga Pradīpikā describes fewer mudrā-s because, it does not include the cleansing of these five elements.

Kriyā-s (cleansing techniques) in the haṭha yoga texts

Date: 1980 | Topic series: Gheraṇḍa Samhitā

1. The Gheraṇḍa Samhitā begins with the "cleansing the pot"—the pot here refers to the body. It describes six kriyā-s and multiple practices under each.

2. The Haṭha Yoga Pradīpikā lists the same six kriyā-s but does not give so many options under each. It recommends that these kriyā-s should be done before pranayama.

3. However, the Haṭha Yoga Pradīpikā (2.36) also says that sages like Yājñavalkya do not approve of these kriyā-s. They are of the opinion that pranayama itself can cleanse the body.

4. If we examine the kriyā-s we can see that, in these days, the disadvantages of these kriyā-s are more than their advantages.

5. The sages like Yājñavalkya are of the opinion that these kriyā-s should be done only by those who need to balance the doshas (vāta, pitta, kapha). Therefore, the Yoga Yājñavalkya does not contain these kriyā-s.

6. Some people are connecting these kriyā-s to the kriyā-yoga of Patanjali. They are different. But the practice of tapas under the kriyā-yoga of Patanjali includes control over food and pranayama practice. This will itself balance the doṣa-s.

Viparīta karaṇī mudrā: practice pointers

Date: 1976 | Topic series: Haṭha Yoga Pradīpikā

1. Viparīta karaṇī mudrā is connected with both headstand and shoulderstand.

2. We must understand the difference between asana and mudrā. Through mudrā, we experience lightness in the body. Because the impurities in the body are removed, the flow of prāṇa is altered. Mudrā should be done with a focused mind, and it will in turn increase our mental steadiness.

3. Another meaning of mudrā is "that which gives us happiness." By focusing the mind, it creates a pleasant experience. This will help lead us to samādhi.

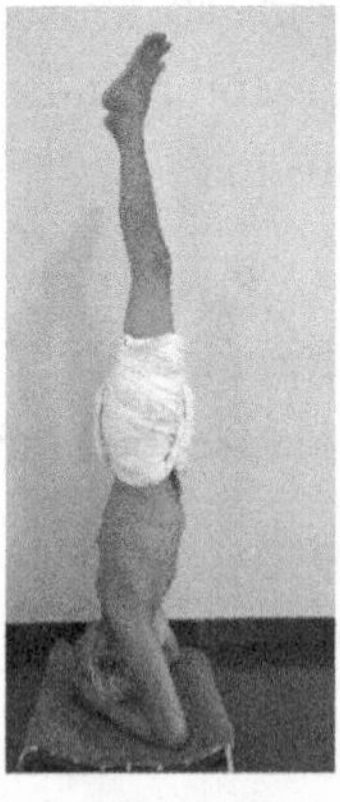
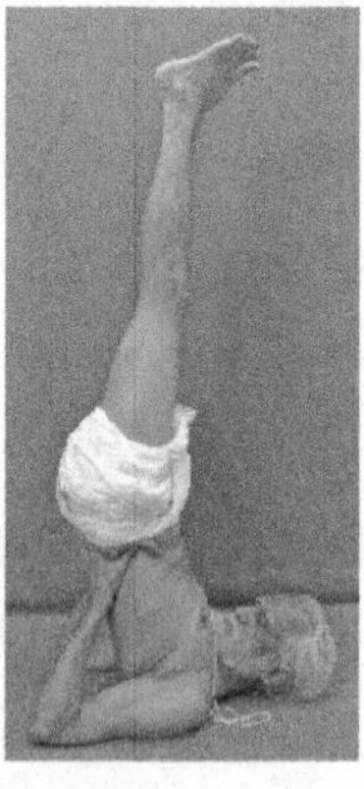

4. Importantly, when you practice viparīta karaṇī mudrā, it should not create pain or discomfort in the body because that will disturb the mind. Therefore, you must practice it gradually, in steps.

5. Headstand is known variously as śīrṣasana, kapālāsana, and bramhaśīrṣāsana. In this asana, first get used to doing long exhale. Then you should practice suspension after exhale.

6. For example, first practice 10 seconds exhale. Then do 10 seconds exhale plus 10 seconds suspension after exhale. Then do 10 seconds inhale, 10 seconds exhale, and 10 seconds suspension after exhale. After this, practice hold after inhale and see how long you can hold the breath. You can start with 5 seconds, for example. Always develop the practice in steps.

7. Headstand is not wise in pregnancy. Especially in later months, headstand should not be practiced.

8. When you do headstand, the flow of prāṇa and the place of apāna change.

9. In shoulderstand, the length of your breath will be shorter. For example, you can do 5 seconds inhale and 10 seconds exhale without any holding (5-0-10-0). Then you can do 5 seconds inhale, 10 seconds exhale, and 5 seconds suspension after exhale (5-0-10-5). Then you can introduce 5 seconds hold after inhale (5-5-10-5). If you do too much hold after inhalation in shoulderstand, you may develop pain in the chest.

3 / *Pranayama*

The traditional texts compare sages to fire. When you see a burning fire, it brings about a feeling in you that you cannot approach it without care. It has too much power, radiance.

You could understand this if you saw Krishnamacharya—he was a modern example. In 1979, he was 91 years old. It was at this time that he gave me detailed classes on pranayama. He was fully fit and mentally sharp.

You could never approach Krishnamacharya casually. Your dress, speech, behavior, posture, body language all had to be thoughtful and respectful. It was not that he was egoistic or demanded it. There was such an extraordinary presence and radiance in him that it would feel inappropriate and discordant otherwise. If you were scattered or casual, you would not fit in his presence. He would, rightly, accept to spend time and energy to teach you only if you showed the proper seriousness, and that included all aspects of yourself.

It was not easy to consider asking a person like him a question. It would be like asking the sun to rise a little sooner so that I can have some light in my room. The right attitude is to be patient in the presence of the sun as it will anyway light up the whole earth and the room with full brightness. You would need to think several times before venturing to ask him anything: Is this question necessary? Am I pressing myself forward unnecessarily as a mark of my lack of confidence in him? He teaches with so much depth and comprehensiveness anyway—will he address this topic as we go along? Do I really understand the subject well enough to ask this question?

In 1979 I had known him for around 8 years, so I could approach him with more confidence. I could begin to ask him some questions too—I knew what would be relevant to ask, and he understood me well enough to accept my sincerity and dedication.

I requested him to teach me pranayama in-depth, because I had to deliver a program on pranayama in Europe soon. I knew that he was extremely keen that only sound yoga should be propagated, so it was the right time, as teacher and student, for me to ask.

He agreed and spent several months giving me in-depth classes on pranayama then. In fact, he took just four sūtra-s from the Yoga Sūtra on pranayama and took a couple of months to cover just that section.

Krishnamacharya's presentation of pranayama is unique. These insights based on his practice do not exist as is in the ancient texts and as far as I have come across, not like this in the presentation of any other teacher of his era.

He told me at this time, "You should not say that you are Krishnamacharya's student, and then go around teaching these subjects incorrectly. Learn and practice correctly and then only teach." He felt strongly that it was the responsibility of the teacher to properly guide the student. This was also why he was extremely selective in accepting long-term students: it was vitally important to him that yoga should be passed on properly. He would never compromise on that.

Understanding prāṇa, the foundation of life

Date: 1973 | Topic series: Praśna Upaniṣad

1. The Praśna Upaniṣad answers several important questions about prāṇa. It also gives us the details of meditation with OM. First, we will look at the topic of prāṇa.

2. An important Vedic verse says "Prāṇa protects the universe."[43] The traditional interpretation of the word prāṇa there is that it refers to the Divine. We can also take this verse to mean that the universe here refers to our body. "The prāṇa within us protects our body." In many places in the classical texts, the word prāṇa is used to refer to the air outside as well as the functions inside of us. We should not confuse the two.

3. Vyāsa notes in the Yoga Sūtra (3.15) that prāṇa is an unseen aspect of ourselves. In the sacred thread ritual, when the young boy is initiated into the Gāyatrī mantra and the rituals of sandhyāvandana, a question is asked, "What is the purpose of this?" And the answer given is, "So that I may know the prāṇa." Thus, the inner purpose of these practices of mantra and ritual is to reveal our prāṇa to us.

4. Prāṇa is the foundation of life, but it is not conscious in itself. That function is in the mind. Prāṇa is independent and also subservient. It is independent in carrying out life functions, but it can also be controlled by the mind.

5. When the flow of prāṇa in the body is appropriate, it will protect our health. When it is not okay, it will consume us.[44] The way to maintain appropriate flow of prāṇa is pranayama.

6. The Bhagavad Gita (6.17) says, to go beyond suffering, the yogi must have appropriate diet, activities, and sleep. This will keep our prāṇa flowing well and protect our health. The Haṭha Yoga Pradīpikā (2.16) cautions that by the inappropriate practice of

---

[43] "prāṇo rakṣati viśvamejat" says the Taittiriya Bramhana.

[44] He uses the Sanskrit words *rakṣaṇa*, to protect, and *bhakṣaṇa*, to eat or consume.

yoga, all diseases will arise, through creating inappropriate flow of prāṇa.

7. By practicing pranayama with unequal lengths of inhale, exhale, and holding, we can achieve wellbeing. By practicing pranayama with equal lengths of inhale, exhale, and holding, we can achieve spiritual progress.[45]

Origin of prāṇa

Date: 1973 | Topic series: Praśna Upaniṣad

This session is based on detailed studies of Chapter 3 of the Praśna Upaniṣad.

1. How is prāṇa formed? How does prāṇa enter the body? After joining the body, and being firmly rooted in the body in five divisions, why does the prāṇa leave the body? What is the connection between the air outside and the prāṇa inside? What is the relationship between prāṇa and consciousness?
2. Prāṇa is born from the ātma (consciousness). The word ātma here should be taken to mean the Divine consciousness. Just as a person's shadow is inseparable from him, similarly, prāṇa is the shadow of consciousness.
3. Mind and prāṇa arise along with consciousness—these cannot be separated. Similar to prāṇa, our mind also pervades our body. We call the mind the power of choice or will (icchā-śakti) and the power of function or action (kriyā-śakti).[46]

---

[45] He refers to sama-vṛtti and viṣama-vṛtti pranayama.

[46] The power of choice or will is termed icchā-śakti in Sanskrit. The power of function or action is termed kriyā-śakti.

4. Because we cannot separate the function of prāṇa and mind, to bring stillness to the mind, we must bring the prāṇa to quietness. Since prāṇa is responsible for the functioning of the senses and the body, we need to control the prāṇa in order to control the mind. This is why we give so much importance to pranayama.

5. If we protect our prāṇa wisely, our life force will remain in our body for a long time (we will have a long life).

6. This Upaniṣad uses the metaphor of shadow. This is for a reason. Shadow is darkness. It is the clouding of avidyā.[47] We do actions because of this avidyā, and because of that, we experience the resulting bondage (as explained in the Yoga Sūtra 2.13).

7. Just as a king tells his officials, "You be here. You be there. Govern these regions, perform these duties," similarly, the main prāṇa orders its divisions to be in regions of the body and perform their respective functions.

8. The air outside is connected to our prāṇa inside. The Divine is in both of them.

9. The prāṇa is principally in our heart region in our body. From that heart region, 101 nāḍi-s arise. Consciousness is also located there.

10. At the time of death, if the prāṇa and consciousness leaves the body through the suṣumnā nāḍī, the yogi attains mokṣa.[48]

---

[47] Avidyā is the root of bondage and suffering as explained in the Yoga Sūtra (2.3-9).

[48] Permanent freedom from suffering and the cycle of birth and death.

Strengthening apāna: postures and breathing

Date: 1973 | Topic series: Praśna Upaniṣad

1. When the function of apāna (elimination function, lower abdomen and pelvis) becomes weak, we can strengthen it.
2. Try dvipādapīṭham (bridge) in this way: First, pull the lower abdomen in, then hold for 2 seconds, and then lift the hips. If this is too difficult, do the lifting movement on exhalation (without the holding). You can also stay in dvipādapīṭham (bridge) and lift one leg at a time.
3. Exhalation and holding after exhalation will strengthen weak apāna function.
4. You can also do ūrdhvaprasṛtrapādasana (lifting the legs, lying on the back) on hold after exhalation. Even if the hips lift up a little, that is okay.
5. If there is constipation too, take more oily and moist food. If you take fruits, eat them, do not just drink the juice.
6. If there is excess gas, do mahāmudrā with normal inhale and long exhale. Ensure that the lower abdomen moves in deeply on exhale.
7. To join the apāna with the earth (to strengthen the downward flow), do upaviṣṭakoṇāsana (seated forward bend with knees bent and legs apart) with long exhale and long inhale. Bend forwards as much as possible. Similarly, baddha koṇāsana (seated forward bend with knees bent and legs apart) should be also be done with hold after exhale.
8. If apāna is aggravated during your practice, your chest may hurt. Be careful to not strain the apāna function.
9. To strengthen prāṇa function, hold after inhalation can help.

10. To help with difficulty in falling asleep, practice pratiloma ujjayi with holding after inhale and exhale.

Pranayama defined in the Yoga Sūtra

Date: 1979 | Topic series: Pranayama

This lecture is about Yoga Sūtra 2.49.[49]

1. Why do we need pranayama? Vyāsa has explained that one is unaffected by pairs of opposites (heat, cold etc.) through the practice of asana. But if we do not practice pranayama, we will not have a long life. For this, lengthening the breath is important.

2. Times have changed now, so the teaching methods also may have to be a little different. In the traditional times, mantra was always combined with pranayama, and the mantra used was OM. But let that be and let us come to the sūtra.

3. The basic meaning of this sūtra is, "After you have mastered asana, the normal flow of inhale and exhale should be modified." The word gati here meaning "normal flow" refers to the usual short breath. The word viccheda, typically meaning "to interrupt," means that we should change that habitual flow.

4. How do we change this flow of breath that is usually short? By making the breath longer. This is the meaning of the word āyāma in prāṇāyāma.

5. A newborn child has a much faster breath maybe 40 breaths per minute. That breathing rate then gradually decreases.

---

[49] "tasmin sati śvāsa-praśvāsayoḥ gati-viccedaḥ prāṇāyāṁaḥ" meaning "When asana has been mastered, pausing the flow of inhalation and exhalation is pranayama."

6. Our breath is affected by many factors. For example, by abusing our senses. Traveling here and there. Undisciplined food habits. Irregular activities.

7. In asana, our breath varies with the posture we are in. But in pranayama, we try to maintain our breath steady, unchanging.

8. Vyāsa's commentary defines inhalation as sipping or drawing the air in from outside. He defines exhalation as expelling the air from inside, that is in the lungs, to the outside.

9. Stopping the flow of both, that is inhalation and exhalation, is pranayama. Vyāsa uses the word "absence" here. This word "absence" here does not mean to minimize or have a little of. It means that there is no flow, it is completely absent.

Three types of pranayama in Yoga Sūtra

Date: 1979 | Topic series: Pranayama

This lecture is about the Yoga Sūtra 2.50.[50]

1. The three types of pranayama are: One, to stop the breath after exhaling. Two, to stop the breath after inhaling. Three, to stop the breath at any point, without a deep inhale or exhale (stambha vṛtti prāṇāyāma).

2. By practicing these three types of prāṇāyāma, the unseen prāṇā becomes seen or accessible to us, through a place in the body, duration, and number. By this, our breath also becomes longer and subtler.

---

[50] "bāhya-ābhyantara-stambha-vṛttiḥ deśa-kāla-saṃkhyābhiḥ paridṛṣṭaḥ dīrgha-sūkṣmaḥ" meaning "By the practice of pausing the breath after exhale, inhale, and with a natural breath, watching over with place, duration, and number, it becomes long and subtle."

3. Here, the vṛtti or "activity" mentioned in the sūtra refers to the action of pausing the breath after exhalation, after inhalation, or without doing either.
4. The words dīrgha and sūkṣma meaning "long" and "subtle" refer to the flow of the inhalations and exhalation.
5. In the old days, we used to place a piece of cotton fluff near the nostrils and see how much it moved with the breath, to assess how long and subtle the breath had become with practice.
6. Vyāsa's commentary gives the example of a drop of water on a hot pan shrinking from all sides. This is to explain the third type of pranayama that is done without specifically inhaling or exhaling (stambha-vṛtti prāṇāyāma).
7. Because there is neither inhale nor exhale, the breath simply subsides (shrinks) in place. This is what the Yoga Yājñavalkya refers to by saying that the scattering of the prāṇa decreases from 108 aṅgula-s to 96 aṅgula-s.[51]
8. When you practice this stambha-vṛtti prāṇāyāma, ensure that you take some normal breaths in between.

Three factors that delineate the experience of prāṇa

Date: 1979 | Topic series: Pranayama

This lecture continues the explanation of Yoga Sūtra 2.50.[52]

---

[51] Aṅgula is a traditional personalized unit of measurement. Three aṅgula-s equal the span of our four fingers held together (excluding the thumb).

[52] See the footnote under the previous lecture.

1. By the practice of these prāṇāyāma-s, the flow of prāṇa becomes "seen" to us. This is the import of the word paridṛṣṭa in the sūtra. To "see" prāṇa means that we experience it in our body.
2. This experience of prāṇa is delineated by three factors in the practice: place, time, and number. The third variable, number, is under the second, time.
3. The first factor is place (deśa). We can experience prāṇa in different locations in our body. That is, we can know, "I experience the prāṇa in this way in this region of my body."
4. Traditionally, there are several useful places that we can use to experience prāṇa in our body. This will be explained later.
5. The second factor is the duration (kāla): how long this experience of prāṇa can be sustained. Vyāsa has not specified the duration one should do these pranayama-s for.
6. Since we are doing hold after inhale and exhale in these practices, in modern times especially, we should take the pulse and ensure it is steady and does not increase too much. The person should not become breathless. Always increase the duration of pranayama gradually.
7. In the olden days, the duration of pranayama was measured using mantra. Gāyatrī mantra or OM were used.
8. The third factor is number of rounds (saṅkhyā). Vyāsa's commentary does not specify a particular number.

Orderly steps to increase breath control in pranayama

Date: 1979 | Topic series: Pranayama

This lecture continues the explanation of Yoga Sūtra 2.50. Vyāsa's commentary only indicates this practice structure. Sri Krishnamacharya has expanded on it to give us these useful pathways.

1. The Sanskrit word udghāta used in the commentaries to mean the "upward push" that you feel when you need to breathe. It is the feeling that "I cannot retain the breath inside me any longer." Or "I cannot keep the breath pushed outside." When you do pranayama, you need to find out how long it takes for this feeling to arise in you.

2. This is not discovered in one breath. You should find how long this is for you over many rounds of breath.

3. Three types of pranayama have been mentioned in the sūtra-s, involving pausing the breath after exhale, after inhale, and without the effort of either.

4. However, the starting point of pranayama practice is indicated in Vyāsa's commentary under the section on number of rounds (saṅkhyā). He mentions three levels of intensity: mild, moderate, and intense.

5. Commentators relate these three levels to the length of the count of breath. For example, as 36 seconds, 72 seconds, and 108 seconds.

6. But this is not possible nowadays. You can start with 5 seconds, 8 seconds, 12 seconds for mild, moderate, and intense levels for ordinary practitioners. The practitioner must find out how many rounds he can do with these counts.

7. If you use a mantra in your mind to measure the length of breath, you will not exceed your limits.
8. These three levels that Vyāsa mentions are not related only to the length of the breath. There is also a krama (order) in types of pranayama practice.
9. Vyāsa first mentions inhale and exhale. So, we should take that to be the mild level. We begin with long exhale and long inhale and find when udghāta arises in us.
10. If we don't pay close attention to udghāta arising, we cannot develop long and subtle breath.
11. We should do the pranayama-s in the order indicated in the sūtra itself: first hold after exhale, and then hold after inhale, and then stopping without effort of inhale or exhale.
12. So, the second level (moderate), is to practice hold after exhale and hold after inhale and watch for the arising of udghāta.
13. The third level (intense) is stopping without fully inhaling or exhaling (stambha vṛtti pranayama).

Fourth pranayama: breathing in steps and effortless breath

Date: 1979 | Topic series: Pranayama

This lecture is about the Yoga Sūtra 2.51.[53]

---

[53] "bāhya-ābhyantara-viṣaya-ākṣepī caturthaḥ" meaning "The fourth [pranayama] is beyond external and internal aspects (unlike the earlier pranayama-s)."

1. The fourth pranayama is beyond the place, time, and rounds that delineate the earlier three pranayama-s.
2. Vyāsa explains the process as "mastering the ground." This is to be done in steps.
3. First, the breath must become long and subtle. This must be mastered on inhalation and exhalation, and then in various points in the inhale and exhale.
4. When this mastery is achieved, then the fourth pranayama arises. You can then pause the breath effortlessly at any point, without the need to use the place, time, and rounds to control it.
5. To achieve the mastery of the ground, the practice to be used is stepped breathing. Inhale partially, hold, inhale a little more, hold, inhale a little more, hold. Similarly, exhale a little, hold, exhale a little more, hold, exhale a little more, hold.
6. In the order of progression, you must first master stepped exhale separately. At this phase, let your inhale be long and smooth, but do not practice stepped inhalation at the same time. Then, master stepped inhalation separately. At this time, let your exhale be long and smooth; do not practice stepped exhalation at the same time. Then combine both, doing stepped inhalation and stepped exhalation practices in the same round of breathing.
7. When you hold the breath here, do meditation with a mantra. This will lead to one-pointed focus of the mind.
8. When this focus deepens, later, you will not be aware of the inhaling, exhaling, and holding. It will become effortless. This is when the fourth pranayama arises. This pranayama does not arise only from breath-control ("prāṇa control"); it depends on mind-control as well.

9. To do this carefully in the steps, as mentioned by Vyāsa under the sūtra on viniyoga (3.6), "yoga is your teacher." Your own practice will guide you. You must watch over how your breath is, with attention and progress accordingly. This is similar to other internal practices like vairāgya—only each person knows the degree of desire they feel within themselves.
10. This practice of stepped breathing should be done carefully and gradually. Otherwise, as the Haṭha Yoga Pradīpikā (2.15-16) says, practice beyond limits and inappropriate practice will create health problems.
11. When doing this stepped breathing, use the following deśa (place of inner focus in the body) to assist in the practice. On the exhalation, move your focus from the mūla (base, pelvic floor region) to the center of the eyebrows, in steps. On the inhalation, move your focus from the from the diaphragm to the feet, in steps.

Breathing in steps and control over our five prāṇa-s

Date: 1977 | Topic series: Yoga Sūtra

This lecture is about the Yoga Sūtra 3.39 which explains a particular siddhi (extraordinary ability). This siddhi arises from mastering the function of udāna-vāyu, which underlies the function of drawing in food and water (~swallowing). In this context Sri Krishnamacharya explained the use of stepped breathing, with a special name, vairambha pranayama. Here, the focus is on the inner control of the movement of the breath and life functions. It is also related to the drying through the air element and increase of agni.

1. To control the function of the vāyu-s, nāḍīśodhana pranayama with unequal (specific) ratios of inhalation, exhalation, and breath-holding is important.
2. And within this practice, pausing the breath after exhalation is particularly important.
3. A specific pranayama is crucial in controlling both prāṇa and apāna. It is called "vairambha pranayama."
4. Rambhā means banana. If you cut open the stem of the banana tree, you will see that there are fine threads inside it. Our nāḍi-s (inner body channels) are so fine like that, invisible to our eyes.
5. The inside of the banana stem is also sticky. Similarly, our nāḍi-s also have blockages due to stickiness.
6. Vairambha pranayama removes this excessive stickiness and water component from our nāḍi-s.
7. Inhale for 2 seconds. Hold the breath for 2 seconds. Again, inhale for 2 seconds. Again, hold for 2 seconds.
8. Then, exhale for 2 seconds. Hold the breath for 2 seconds. Again, exhale for 2 seconds. Again, hold for 2 seconds.
9. According to capacity, the practitioner can increase this length of 2 seconds to 3 seconds, and then further. It should be done with krama (logical, appropriate progression).
10. This is a practice that involves breathing in and out in steps.
11. The attention of the mind should be placed on different parts of the lungs while we do this stepped breathing.
12. This practice is recommended in the practice pathway of the Yoga Sūtra. Kapālabhāti is not preferred. The body will shake and stability (sthira) will be lacking.

Pranayama in the traditional Vedic texts

Date: 1979 | Topic series: Pranayama

Pranayama is a part of all the traditional Vedic rituals. Therefore, the ancient texts contain many recommendations on doing pranayama. Here, Krishnamacharya has presented important sayings from traditional sources.

Mantra in pranayama

1. In the ancient days, pranayama was always done with a mantra. The gāyatrī mantra was the usual one used with pranayama.

Equal and unequal ratios in pranayama and their use

2. Bhagavad Gita 5.27 says, "Make the inhalations and exhalations equal and breathe through the nose." This equal breath pranayama (sama vṛtti pranayama) is recommended to steady the mind and also used by the yogi at the time of leaving the body (Bhagavad Gita 8.13).

3. Pranayama with unequal length of the inhale and exhale (viṣama vṛtti pranayama) mentioned in the Bhagavad Gita 4.29 is generally used for wellbeing of the body and in therapy.

Asana, saṅkalpa, pranayama always go together

4. All the Vedic rituals contain some asana, saṅkalpa (~intention), and pranayama. The texts say, "Sit in an asana, state the saṅkalpa, and then start pranayama."

5. The saṅkalpa (intention) regarding pranayama should be clear about "Which technique will I use to make the breath long and subtle? How long and how many rounds?" and that "I will be attentive in this practice."

6. The texts do not always specify the asana to be used. It may vary. Usually, pranayama is done seated. But, in the morning,

pranayama in the rituals may be done standing. At some other points of time, pranayama may be done in the squatting position. It may also be done in one-leg lotus position.

What is pranayama? (Viṣṇu Purāṇa)

7. The Viṣṇu Purāṇa says: "That method by which we bring the vāyu-s such as prāṇa, which are responsible for our life functions, under our control, through appropriate practice—that method is termed pranayama. This pranayama may be practiced with a seed (sa-bīja) and without a seed (a-bīja)."[54]

The third pranayama (Viṣṇu Purāṇa)

8. Prāṇa and apāna are opposing forces. When we control these two by practicing pranayama using hold after exhalation and hold after inhalation, the third type of pranayama arises. Note that these practices should be done carefully.

9. This is equivalent to the fourth pranayama in Yoga Sūtra (2.51). This classification skips over the third type of pranayama (stambha vṛtti pranayama) of the Yoga Sūtra. The Yoga Sūtra splits the stages further to give us a more detailed practice pathway.

Pranayama to meditation (Viṣṇu Purāṇa)

10. Control the prāṇa through pranayama. Then master the senses (indriya-s) through pratyahara. Then steady the mind in a beneficial place. This is the pathway of meditation.

11. To do this, choose one seated posture (such as bhadrāsana), and master that (be steady and comfortable in it).

---

[54] The *seed* here usually refers to a mantra, but it may also refer to using a deity or other specific inner focus of meditation along with the breath control.

12. The inner support of this practice is first the image of the deity (Viṣṇu in this case).

13. Note that the Haṭha Yoga Pradīpikā (3.127) instructs the practitioner to do pranayama always with a focused mind.

Prāṇa removes the impurities in the senses

14. When kindling a fire, we blow air to remove the impurities and enhance the flame. Similarly, by controlling and using the prāṇa, we can kindle the inner fire and remove all the impurities in the senses. (Manu)

In praise of pranayama

15. If we do pranayama at sun rise, with inhalation, exhalation, and holding, all the impurities because of actions in body, mind, and speech are destroyed and scattered like dust. (Samvarta Maharshi)

Pranayama as cleansing, done with mantra

16. First cleanse the body externally with bathing etc. Then, to cleanse the body internally, do pranayama.

17. How should this pranayama be? It should be done with the 7-part gāyatrī mantra, with OM, with equal breath (equal inhalation, holding and exhalation). (Yājñavalkya Saṃhitā)[55]

All these traditional practices should be done with pranayama

18. Pūja (worship), japa (meditation with mantra), homa (Vedic rituals with offerings in a fire), veda-adhyayana (Vedic chanting), śrāddha (rituals after demise), snāna (bathing), dāna (charity), dhyāna (meditation), arghya-pradāna (one of the offerings in the rituals of sandhyāvandana): all these should be done with

---

[55] This text is not the Yoga Yājñavalkya. It is the Yājñavalkya Smṛti.

pranayama, three times, and each round of pranayama should have inhale, holding and exhale.

Pranayama should be done with the finger position of mṛgi-mudrā

19. Use the thumb, ring finger, and little finger during pranayama. Leave out the middle finger and the index finger. Pranayama will yield benefit only when done this way. (Karma Pradīpa)

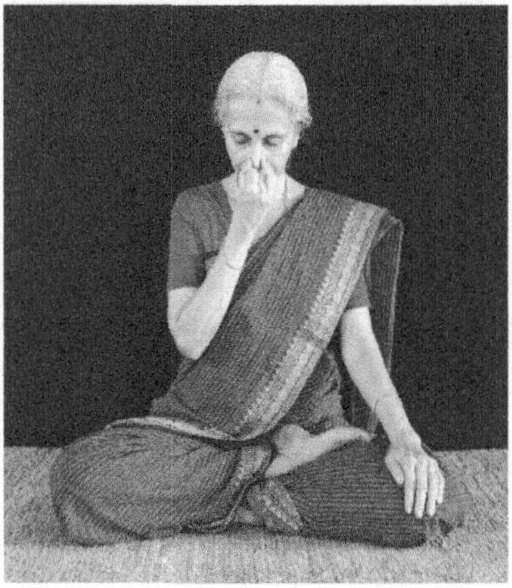
Pranayama with mṛgi mudrā

Definition of pranayama

20. Prāṇa is the force that supports our body from within. (It is not the air from outside.) When we bring it under our control, by making it long and subtle, that is called pranayama. This is of two types: with and without meditation (using a mantra).[56] (Nāradīya Samhitā)

21. You can also use this classification for asana, depending on whether you do it with an inner meditation focus or not.

22. If you neither draw the breath in or out, this is called śūnyaka pranayama or kevala kumbhaka.[57]

---

[56] This is termed agarbha and sagarbha—pregnant with the seed of a mantra or not.

[57] Śūnya = "devoid of," meaning devoid of the effort inhale and exhale. Kevala kumbhaka = "only holding," referring to the fourth pranayama of Yoga Sūtra 2.51.

Breathe slowly through the nose in pranayama

23. Pranayama involves inhale, holding, and exhalation. Filling the air inside the body by drawing it in through the nose is the inhalation. Holding is to keep that air without movement inside. Releasing the air through the nose is exhalation. Do meditation with the mantra when holding (as concentration is maximum then). Always release the air slowly through the nose, never rapidly. The body should not shake.

24. Breathe the air in slowly for 12 counts through the left nostril and fill the lungs. Focus your eyes on the tip of the nose and meditate. Exhale slowly. (Yājñavalkya Saṃhitā)

The limit and signs of effective breath holding

25. The limit of holding the breath is when you feel it until the tip of your hairs and the circulation in your nails. However, the next exhalation should remain controlled and long. If you are able to sustain such a breath, it fully expands inside the body. This increases the metabolism (~abdominal fire). Because of this, the water in the body tends to come out, hence the practitioner begins to perspire. Together, these actions of the air, fire, and water cleanse the body from within.

Combining pranayama and mantra meditation

Date: 1979 | Topic series: Pranayama

1. First bring the gāyatrī mantra to mind. Then wash the hands and legs, cleansing the body externally.

2. Sit in a stable asana, facing east. Then cleanse yourself internally using ācamana (a ritual with sips of water combined with mantra chanting).

3. Then begin pranayama. The pranayama should be done with the 7-part gāyatrī mantra.

4. Follow this with meditation on the gāyatrī mantra. In this meditation, the gāyatrī mantra should be preceded with OM and followed by OM. That is the gāyatrī mantra should be enclosed in the sound of OM.

5. You can do 12 rounds of pranayama followed by 12 rounds of mantra meditation. This duration and repetitions can be modified to suit the capacity of the practitioner.

4 / Mind & Meditation

The foundation of yoga is the capacity to focus our attention calmly. This was a teaching that Krishnamacharya emphasized, always. He himself was an example par excellence of this.

Meditation and mindfulness are a part of all the other limbs and practices of yoga. All asana in his teaching involved steady, mindful movement. One should always have focus when doing asana. For instance, the gaze should usually be toward the heart center, and attention should be placed within.

You would never see him moving in a scattered manner. If he sat in one place, he would remain still. No wandering of the mind, and hence no restlessness of the body.

Further, asana always incorporated attentive breathing. And pranayama was a practice of absorption in the breath.

At the center of his meditation and mindfulness practice was his devotion to the Divine. From morning to night, the connection to the Divine in the heart center and in all activities was an anchor of his life. This was also an anchor for meditation.

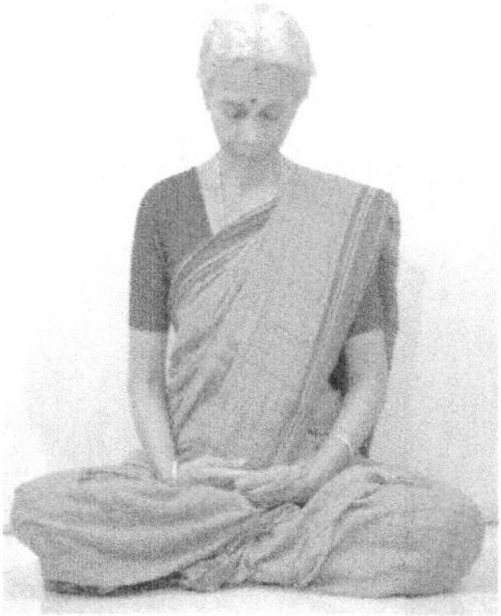

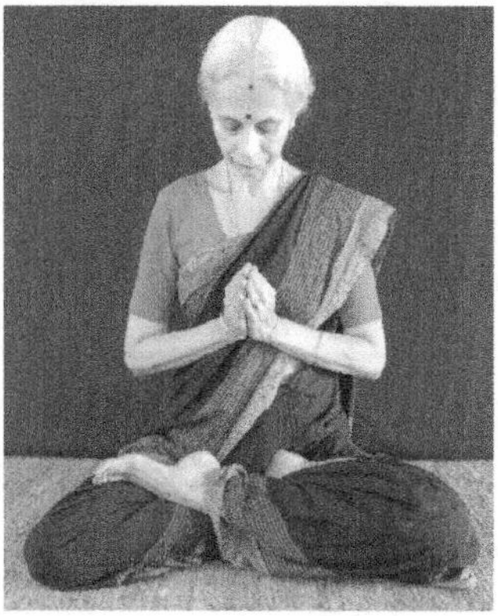

Ritual in the form of sandhyāvandana and puja (worship of the Divine) was a thread in his life every day. While many people do these mechanically, Krishnamacharya did them with complete attention, not just as actions, but as absorption and transformation.

He used to explain that we can do asana and pranayama also as devotional meditation: "Offer the breath to the Divine, just as you offer a flower when you do puja."

Mantra was a background of his life. No unnecessary speech crossed his lips if he could avoid it. Instead, he would repeat his mantra in his mind. Similarly, Vedic chanting was also a time of total attention: to the sound and the meaning.

We often speak of mindfulness and meditation, but we rarely find someone in life making it an integral part of their life. Krishnamacharya was a striking example of embodying mindfulness through yoga and devotion.

Meditation on the Divine using the mantra OM

Date: 1980 | Topic series: Yoga Sūtra

This lecture is about the Yoga Sūtra 1.27.[58]

1. Because the transcendental Divine does not have a physical form, it is signified by a sound. That sound is OM, also known as praṇava.
2. The root meaning of the word praṇava implies "to honor or praise well."

---

[58] "tasya vācakaḥ praṇavaḥ" meaning "The signifier of the Divine, Īśvara, is the mantra OM."

3. Here, we must understand that to "honor" the Divine is to meditate on the Divine.
4. The sound used here is OM. The object or experience the sound refers to is the Divine.
5. In this context, the connection between the word and the object, between OM and the Divine, is indivisible, eternal.
6. In the commentary on mīmāṁsā (Śābara Bhāṣya), it is explained that the sound brings the object to mind. This enables us to experience, to see, the object clearly.
7. Here, through the practice of the mantra OM, what we experience clearly is our own consciousness.
8. This experience is internal to us; this is explained in the next sūtra.
9. Practically, the sound of OM helps us keep the recall of Īśvara in our mind. This will lead to one-pointed focus of mind.
10. If we wish to develop such focus, we should use the sound of OM aloud with a length of three counts (~seconds) in meditation.
11. In puja (worship and rituals), we should use OM with a length of two counts.
12. In mental japa (meditation with the mantra silently in the mind), we should use OM with a length of one count.
13. When meditating with a mantra, we must do so with the recall of the experience (artha) or object that the mantra signifies. This is svādhyāya.
14. Vyāsa says this in his commentary: Through svādhyāya, the practice of yoga grows, and through yoga, the practice of svādhyāya is deepened. This will lead to the illumination of the experience of the Divine.

Pausing the breath after exhale

Date: 1980 | Topic series: Yoga Sūtra

This lecture is about the Yoga Sūtra 1.34.[59]

1. Our body has nine openings or doors. The Bhagavad Gita (5.13) mentions this.
2. These doors are the ways by which our energy is scattered. This in turn can lead to unsteadiness and weakness of the mind.
3. Chapter 1 of the Yoga Sūtra lists nine means of steadying and clearing the mind.
4. Chapter 2 of the Yoga Sūtra says that the scattering of the mind can be managed through pranayama.
5. The word used here to denote exhalation is pracchardana—the root of this word has the meaning "vomiting." The reason for the choice of this word is: the practice here entails completely expelling the air by a long exhale.
6. The second word in the practice component is vidhāraṇa, which means "to hold firmly." This is not referring just to the breath. It implies holding the mind firmly.
7. The mind naturally stops after exhale. At that time, use OM mantra, and place the mind on the inner experience of the Divine. This is mentioned in the Bhagavad Gita (8.13).
8. The movement of the cakras and exhalation are connected. By using a long exhalation, it is possible to transcend (take the prāṇa and awareness up and beyond) the six lower cakras.

---

[59] "pracchardana-vidhāraṇābhyāṃ vā prāṇasya" meaning "By pausing the breath after exhalation, the mind becomes calm and clear."

9. Going beyond the six cakras in haṭha yoga is equivalent in the Upaniṣads to going beyond the six waves of bondage (desire, anger, greed, delusion, pride, envy).[60]

10. Our inhale and exhale are also related to the aspects of the buddhi in Sāṁkhya of ethics, knowledge, non-attachment, and power.[61]

11. This sūtra does not tell us in which asanas this should be practiced. Except in the ritual of sandhyāvandana, normally pranayama is done in a seated posture.

12. By the practice of inhale, long exhale, and holding after exhale, our body becomes lighter and our mind, steadier.

13. Do not force the inhale or exhale through blocked nostrils in pranayama. Asana will help you to clear the nostrils.

14. Gāyatrī mantra can be useful in lengthening the exhale. Use the parts of the gāyatrī mantra in steps to add length.

15. When you do pranayama, try to seal the senses.

---

[60] These are well-known as the ṣaḍ-ūrmi: kāma, krodha, lobha, moha, mada, mātsarya.

[61] The buddhi-bhāva-s are dharma, jñāna, vairāgya, aiśvarya, and their four opposites.

Practicing the subtle experience of the senses

Date: 1980 | Topic series: Yoga Sūtra

This lecture is about the Yoga Sūtra 1.35.[62]

1. This is one of the means to steady the mind. Here, the word "activity" refers to the activities of our mind (citta).
2. Our mind connects with objects through the senses. By "object," we mean sight, sound, touch, taste, smell.
3. If we can bring the subtle experience of these senses to our awareness, our mind will stay steady there.
4. For example, if we close our ears and practice nādānusandhāna (~listening to the inner sound), our mind becomes absorbed in that subtle sound. The Haṭha Yoga Pradīpikā expands on this practice.
5. Place a drop of honey on the tip of your tongue, feel that sweetness, and then focus your mind on the foundation of that sensation.
6. You can do a similar practice for each of the other senses too.
7. By this practice, steadiness of the mind arises. The signs of this steadiness of mind that arise before that are explained in the Śvetāśvatara Upaniṣad (2.11): snowflakes, smoke, sun, wind, fire, fireflies, lightning, crystals, and the moon.
8. These are not material or gross objects that we see in the world outside. These are the inner illuminations of the senses manifesting in these forms.

---

[62] "viṣayavatī vā pravṛttiḥ utpannā manasaḥ sthiti-nibandhinī" meaning "By the experience born of this special focus e.g., on the tip of the nose, the mind is bound."

9. Externally the signs are lightness and healthiness of the body, diminishing desire, clear complexion, pleasantness of voice, sweet odor, and reduced excretions. (Śvetāśvatara Upaniṣad 2.13)

10. Similarly, gazing at the sun and the moon can be useful for steadying the mind. This said, we must question whether we need to do these practices. We have many vāsana-s[63] inside us that may manifest as we have these subtle experiences, and we may be trapped by them. It is better to follow the teachings of the great sages and those who have practiced the classical and safer pathways.[64]

"I" feeling and the heart lotus: the ancient pathway

Date: 1980 | Topic series: Yoga Sūtra

This lecture is about the Yoga Sūtra 1.36.[65]

1. The state referred to here is the experience of being free of all unhappiness or suffering. It is an illuminated experience.

2. The place of meditation in this sūtra is the "heart lotus." Here the word used refers to a lotus that is facing downward and has not yet bloomed.

---

[63] Vāsana-s are the samskāra-s or stored patterns of pleasure and suffering that bind us.

[64] "Follow the ācārya-s, śāstra-s, and īśvara praṇidhāna."

[65] "viśokā vā jyotiṣmatī" meaning "By meditation on light in the heart lotus, all suffering is removed."

3. Where is this place of the heart lotus? It is mentioned in the Nārāyaṇa Upaniṣad: 12 aṅgula-s above the navel and 12 aṅgula-s below the pit of the throat.

4. How to practice this? Use holding after exhale, with the three bandhas. This will turn the heart lotus to face upward.

5. Then you must bring awareness to this place of the heart lotus and hold it steady there. In sūtra 3.1 on dhāraṇā, Vyāsa mentions the heart lotus as one of the preferred places to hold our attention steady. You cannot succeed in this practice without the capacity for stable attention (dhāraṇā).

6. The Chāndogya Upaniṣad (8.1.1) refers to the same place in the heart lotus and this practice.

7. 101 nāḍī-s (subtle channels) are connected with the heart lotus as mentioned in the Praśna Upaniṣad (3.6). Among those one nāḍī travels upward from the heart center.

8. In the sound OM, there are three syllables, Aa, Uu, and Mm. Among these, Aa denotes the illumination of the waking state. Here sattva is dominant. Uu refers to the dreaming state. Here rajas is dominant. Mm refers to the state of deep sleep. Here tamas is dominant.

9. The threads of these three gunas (the experiences of all three states) are a part of this nāḍī leading upward from the heart center.

10. By this practice (focus with holding after exhale as mentioned earlier), the experience of sattva expands in the heart lotus and this nāḍī. At that time, the mind becomes like the sky illuminated by the sun.

11. At this point, we see the nature of asmitā (the "I" experience) clearly.[66]

12. Just as the body become stable through asana, the mind becomes totally steady through this practice.

Samādhi and its connection with prāṇa and pranayama

Date: 1977 | Topic series: Yoga Sūtra

This lecture is about the Yoga Sūtra 3.3. This sūtra defines samādhi. He explained this sūtra over several days.[67]

Following sage Vyāsa's commentary, Sri Krishnamacharya first explains the sūtra. Then he adds his insights.

1. When one is in samādhi, there is no external awareness. There is only inner awareness.

2. The Māṇḍūkya Upaniṣad has a detailed explanation of this inner awareness.[68]

3. In dhyāna (the earlier step), there are three components: the place of focus, the object of focus, and the mind. When all these three become one, and the activity in the citta appears to have

---

[66]This practice and its description by the ancient yogis is important. It has deep insight into the body-mind connection.

[67] "tadeva artha-mātra-nirbhāsaṁ svarūpa-śūnyam iva samādhiḥ" meaning "When the experience alone is illuminated, as if the self has ceased to exist, that is samādhi."

[68] The Sanskrit word used in Māṇḍūkya Upaniṣad is antaḥ-prajñā.

stopped, and the feeling that "I am meditating," is gone—that is samādhi.

4. Our mind is like a lake. The objects in the world are like stones. If we toss the stones in the lake, there are many waves. Like that, the objects create waves in the mind because of desire. Our mind becomes deeply content when it is in samādhi. Why? Because the Divine that we are meditating on shines in that state. This is the import of verse 2.55 from the Bhagavad Gita.

5. The mind and prāṇa are stilled at the time of samādhi. They reflect our consciousness. Unless prāṇa is controlled, the mind will not stay still like this. Therefore, pranayama is important.

6. How should we practice pranayama? The Vedic definition of pranayama is that it should be done with the gāyatrī mantra.

7. Pranayama should be done with all three bandha-s. Without uddīyāna-bandha, the diaphragm goes down. Without jalandhara-bandha, chest pain will result. Any retention after inhale should always be done with jalandhara-bandha. Holding after exhale should be done with mūla-bandha.

8. If mūla-bandha is practiced all the time, one needs to be careful. It may result in diarrhea, wet dreams, and kidney trouble.

9. First practice pranayama with equal inhale and exhale, then practice unequal ratios. This is referenced in the Bhagavad Gita, chapters 5 and 4.

Light in the crown cakra, headstand practice, siddha-s

Date: 1977 | Topic series: Yoga Sūtra

This lecture is about the Yoga Sūtra 3.32. This sūtra relates to a special power (siddhi) of being able to see the siddha-s (~celestial beings).

1. The crown of the head is the spot where we find a softness in infants. This is where we rest the head when we do headstand.
2. The Nārāyaṇa Upaniṣad says that there is a flame in the heart center, and in that space, one can experience consciousness through meditation.
3. Similarly, there is light in this space at the crown of the head. This is what Vyāsa's commentary on this sūtra mentions.
4. Siddha-s are said to inhabit the space between the earth and sky. How is this idea connected to our body? The sky is crown chakra at the top of the head. The earth is the rest of the body below. The space between them is the location where this light is experienced.
5. To prepare for this practice, do inner gazing[69] on light, with steady attention. The outer gaze should be toward the center of eyebrows.
6. Try this inner gazing in shoulderstand. Then try this in headstand, yoga mudrā, and yoga nidrā positions.
7. If you continue this practice (samyama), you will begin to see that inner light at the space below the crown of the head. In time, you will transcend that light and experience a vision of the siddha-s.

---

[69] antah-trāṭaka dhāraṇā is the term used.

Why do we not progress in yoga?

Date: 1980 | Topic series: Yoga Sūtra

This lecture is about the Yoga Sūtra 2.10.[70] Here, Sri Krishnamacharya takes a list from the Hitopadeśa (2.5), a famous collection of ancient Sanskrit stories that give general wisdom. In its literal meaning, this verse lists obstacles to achievement in life. He modifies them to make them relevant to achieving progress on the path of yoga and diminishing the kleśa-s.

These kleśa-s[71] stay active because of these common causes.

1. Laziness and postponing our yoga practices.
2. Chasing after sex, physically and through company.
3. Returning to destructive habits, due to the strength of older actions.
4. Excessive attachment to one's own body.
5. Extremes of emotion, including the highs.
6. Giving into the weakness of unnecessary fear.

---

[70] "te pratiprasava-heyaḥ sūkṣmāḥ" meaning "The subtle kleśa-s should be removed through not allowing them to arise."

[71] Yoga Sūtra 2.3-9 lists the kleśa-s and explains them. They are five fundamental misperceptions that cause suffering: avidyā (the field on which the others arise), asmitā (self as non-self), rāga (desire), dveśa (dislike), abhiniveśa (fear).

5 / *Mantra & Rituals*

When I saw Krishnamacharya for the first time in 1971, he was delivering a lecture on sandhyāvandana. It was not the topic that drew me to him—it was his presence.

Later, in a private class, he mentioned, "Someone came with a mental health problem, and I told him to practice sandhyāvandana. That will help." I did not understand at that time how the ritual could help.

In July 1977, he delivered a series of weekly lectures over several months, explaining sandhyāvandana in detail. He explained the structure of the ritual, steps, mantra, bhavana, nyasa, the inner meaning of it all, and more. Then, I began to understand the topic better.

In 1986, I had a series of classes on the topic of rituals itself. He again spoke about sandhyāvandana, but this time in a larger context. Krishnamacharya himself practiced sandhyāvandana every day.

Done with concentration and the full length of pranayama and meditation, it will take around forty-five minutes, to be repeated thrice a day. To make it possible for students in modern times, he also explained which were the most important aspects of the practice that one should focus on, to do it in a shorter duration.

I recall him giving me many practical instructions during that teaching. He told me, "Try it now. Go into utkaṭāsana (squat) position. See how your legs press on your stomach? If you stomach grows, you will not be able to do pranayama in this position. Only if your belly does not grow will you be healthy. This is another reason why you should include pranayama in these positions, like you do in this ritual."

Another instruction was, "When you do this ritual in the morning, you should face the light of the sun. You should glance towards the sun, then lower your gaze. Close your eyes halfway, so you are still experiencing that light. Then do pranayama in this standing position, with meditation."

In 1983-84, he took several hours to explain the gāyatrī mantra and the many aspects of its meaning, practice, and much more. He was kind enough to record these lectures so that this message would not be lost. We have presented the materials here based on those lectures.

Vedic chanting was the practice of longest duration in Krishnamacharya's life. He has said that his father began teaching him Vedic chanting when he was just 5 years old. It was his firm opinion that health of the body, long life, concentration, and clarity of mind would arise from Vedic chanting. He has mentioned this so many times over the years.

Vedic chanting is also a form of pranayama because of the long breath. It can also be used to modulate the length of our breath because the passages have varying numbers of syllables.

I learned Vedic chanting from Krishnamacharya one to one from 1976 to his last days in 1989. Vedic chanting requires focus. He would correct me when I made mistakes. This was one of the reasons why he began recording his classes for me: to ensure that there were no mistakes in Vedic chanting, and later, in transmitting his teachings on other topics. In 1983-84 he gave some detailed lectures on Vedic chanting. He was kind enough to permit recording these lectures too.

In the late years, he had once told me, "Come tomorrow and I will teach you about pūjā—rituals for the traditional worship." The class was somewhat early in the morning, around 8 am. When I arrived, he had a plate in his hand and was eating a dosa. He told me, "You should not eat first and then do the pūjā. I have become and old man now. I am unable to follow all the external disciplines as I used to. But because I am teaching you now after eating, you must not do the same thing. Do not say, 'My guru used to eat before puja,' and skip the disciplines when you practice or teach these subjects!"

A vital reason he used to emphasize rituals and surrender to the Divine was, in his words, "If you only pursue other studies and practice without the right bhāvana (feeling and attitude) and bhakti (devotion and surrender), your ego will increase."

Gāyatrī mantra: introduction, structure, syllables

Date: 1983-1984 | Topic series: Gāyatrī mantra

1. Gāyatrī is a Vedic mantra. Mantra is "that which protects us when we repeat it." This is the general meaning.
2. Gāyatrī mantra is a particular set of syllables that is chanted with specific notes in the morning, afternoon, and evening.
3. We can also understand the gāyatrī in the three parts from the roots of gā, ya, and tra. *Gā* means to chant. *Ya* means to spread, meaning that it fills the body. *Tra* means to protect. When chanted, it spreads throughout our body and protects us.
4. I will explain these briefly: the meaning of the gāyatrī mantra, the form of the gāyatrī deity, how we should meditate using the gāyatrī, and in which places (in the body).
5. The centerpiece (heart) of the gāyatrī mantra has three parts:

   tat savitur vareṇīyam |

   bhargo devasya dhīmahi |

   dhiyo yo naḥ pracodayāt |
6. Each of these three parts has 8 syllables. In total, the mantra has 24 syllables. These 24 syllables indicate the 24 tattva-s of Sāṃkhya.
7. Before the centerpiece of the gāyatrī mantra, OM and three syllables known as vyahṛti-s are added:

OM bhūḥ bhuvaḥ suvaḥ

[followed by the centerpiece]

8. These 24 tattva-s are subject to change. What underlies these 24 tattva-s, that does not change, is OM. That represents the Divine.
9. That Divine is responsible for creation, sustenance, and absorption. The three vyahṛti-s (bhūḥ bhuvaḥ suvaḥ) represent the three worlds.
10. The qualities of that Divine and the purpose of the meditation are in the centerpiece of the mantra.

Meaning of the words of the gāyatrī mantra

Date: 1983-1984 | Topic series: Gāyatrī mantra

tat: That, which we do not see with our eyes, it is beyond the senses.

savituḥ: The Divine that has created and sustains this universe.

vareṇīyam: Most excellent, the greatest. That Divine which will grant us what is best for us.

bhargaḥ: The power that will burn away the impurities in our body and senses.

devasya: The form of that Divine is made of energy, light, power.

dhīmahi: We meditate on that with focused attention. Our mind must become one with that light. This is beyond words; it is to be experienced.

yaḥ: That Divine, that light, of the nature of sound or vibration.

pracodayāt: May it kindle.

dhiyaḥ: The discernment to choose what we should seek, in freedom or material pursuits.

naḥ: In us.

This gāyatrī mantra with these 24 syllables is known as the mahā gāyatrī ("great gāyatrī) or bīja gāyatrī ("seed gāyatrī"). There are variants of the gāyatrī mantra. They are called śākhā gāyatrī-s ("branch gāyatrī"), based on personal deities. The word *pracodayāt* is a key. It is found in all versions of the gāyatrī.

How to meditate on the gāyatrī mantra with a form

Date: 1983-1984 | Topic series: Gāyatrī mantra

1. Traditionally, the gāyatrī is described in a feminine form as a young girl, a woman, and in her elder years—in the morning, afternoon, and evening respectively. They correspond to creation, sustenance, and ending, and to the three Vedas.
2. There is also a single feminine form of the gāyatrī described for meditation at all times. She has 5 faces representing the 5 bhuta-s, 3 eyes representing the sun, moon, and fire. She also bears various ornaments and weapons. In total, these come to 24 in number, equating to the tattva-s of Sāṃkhya.
3. We should first do visualization on the gāyatrī in this form, with the intention that all these elements in us should be purified.
4. We must then meditate on the Divine in our heart region. For this, we first meditate on the Divine in the form of the light of the sun. Remember that the sun is only a representation of the qualities of the Divine.
5. The mantra used is:

   OM bhūḥ bhuvaḥ suvaḥ

   tat savitur vareṇīyam |

bhargo devasya dhīmahi |

dhiyo yo naḥ pracodayāt |

This mantra is called the tripāt gāyatrī (three-part gāyatrī).

How to invoke the gāyatrī mantra in our own body

Date: 1983-1984 | Topic series: Gāyatrī mantra

This was from a private series of lectures that I had with the master on the topic of the gāyatrī mantra.

1. To invoke the gāyatrī in our own body, we must bring the feeling that our body is made of the sound (vibration) of the mantra.
2. For this, various nyāsa-s are used: special placement of the mantra in different parts the body.
3. The mantra used is:

   Oṃ bhūḥ | Oṃ bhuvaḥ | Om̐ suvaḥ | Oṃ mahaḥ | Oṃ janaḥ | Oṃ tapaḥ | Om̐ satyam (*These seven parts are the body of the mantra.)*

   tat savitur vareṇīyam |

   bhargo devasya dhīmahi |

   dhiyo yo naḥ pracodayāt | (*These three lines are the heart of the mantra.)*

   Oṃ āpo jyotī raso'mṛtam bramha bhūrbhuvassuvaroṃ | (*This is the head of the mantra.*)
4. The meditation is done in the heart region.
5. This gāyatrī mantra with the "seven-part body" is used in pranayama.

6. The heart region is the center of our prāṇa. The prāṇa spreads from there to all regions of the body and returns there through five channels, one for each of the divisions of prāṇa.
7. Pranayama should be done with this inner feeling of the flow of prāṇa and with the seven-part gāyatrī mantra. Three parts are below the navel/diaphragm and three parts above the navel/diaphragm.
8. In the practice of sandhyāvandana, "seven-part body" gāyatrī is used in pranayama, and meditation on the gāyatrī mantra is done with the three-part gāyatrī mantra.

Smārta gāyatrī

Date: 1983-1984 | Topic series: Gāyatrī mantra

1. The main gāyatrī mantra is called mahā gāyatrī or bīja gayatrī.[72] To receive the full benefits of that mantra, we must chant it with the correct pronunciation and intonation along with the reflection on its meaning.
2. For this, we must first practice and create the necessary samskāra-s (patterns and connection).
3. We can achieve the same benefits through the smārta gāyatrī mantra. It has no specific intonation and is in verse form:

   yodevassavitāsmākaṃ

   dhiyo dharmādigocarāḥ |

   prerayet tasya yadbhargaḥ

   tadvareṇyaṃ upāsmahe ||

---

[72] Great gāyatrī or seed gāyatrī.

yo devaḥ: That power or light of the Divine.

savitā: The Divine force present inside the sun which is responsible for life.

asmākaṃ: For all of us

dhiyo: Discernment on what is best for us, what we shall do and not do.

dharmadigocarah: In the path of dharma.

prerayet: To kindle.

tasya yad bhargah: The light or the power that removes all the impurities.

tat: That which is beyond sense perception.

vareṇyaṃ: The most worthwhile, excellent.

upāsmahe: Let us meditate with focused mind.

We meditate with focused mind upon the greatest divine power represented by the illumination of the sun. Let it kindle our intellect to follow the path of dharma and purify our mind.

Gāyatrī for personal deities: śākhā gāyatrī-s

Date: 1983-1984 | Topic series: Gāyatrī mantra

1. We can connect our personal deity to the gāyatrī mantra for our practice and meditation.
2. Therefore, there are many versions of the gāyatrī mantra incorporating Śiva, Viṣṇu, Mother Goddess etc.
3. These gāyatrī mantras are called śākhā gāyatrī-s meaning "branch gāyatrī-s."

4. We can even compose our personalized versions of these gāyatrī-s mentioning different forms and qualities of the Divine. However, the key words of the gāyatrī mantra will be retained.

5. The Nārāyaṇa Upaniṣad gives us gāyatrī mantra-s for some of the important traditional deities.

Ritual of sandhyāvandana

Date: 1977-1978 | Topic series: Sandhyāvandana

1. Sandhyāvandana is also called sandhyā upāsana. It is a ritual practice that we must do every day. If we do not, our body and senses become unsteady. Then, the obstacles to yoga practice mentioned in the Yoga Sūtra (1.30) arise. If we do this practice, our willpower grows.

2. You may ask, why are there problems if we don't do this? Actions have results. But inaction also has outcomes. We will end up doing other actions (karma), that will cover our clarity (prajñā). Our consciousness is covered by the prakṛti—that is our actions and the latent impressions of those actions. If we do not practice sandhyāvandana, this covering[73] is not removed.

3. Sandhi means junction. What junction do we refer to here? It is a change of time: when the sun rises, when the sun reaches a peak, and when the sun sets. We offer our salutations at each of these times.

---

[73] Avidyā as mentioned in the Yoga Sūtra.

4. Keep in mind that the external sun in space is only a representation[74] here. What we really meditate on is the Divine in our heart space.
5. The intention of this meditation with a salutation to the sun is the request, "Remove these coverings (avidyā) in me. Show me the right path and lead me to a state of peace."
6. This is the brief meaning, the essence of the gāyatrī mantra. From this meditation, we become a new person—we recreate ourselves, body, senses, and mind.
7. The internal transformations from this meditation may not be fully visible outside. As Patanjali says in 3.15, there are changes that are invisible or hidden. But there is no doubt that these transformations will happen if we practice.
8. The two important practices in sandhyāvandana are pranayama and meditation with gāyatrī mantra.
9. Sandhyāvandana can be done with Vedic mantras or with tāntric mantras[75] or even just in the mind through bhāvana.
10. This practice of sandhyāvandana is not classified as tamasic or rajasic. It is to be done always and is therefore only sattvic.
11. Nowadays, people ask who should do this. The answer is, everyone should do this, all men and women.

---

[74] The word used is *pratīka* used to refer to another object or experience which has similar qualities, and hence represents the other object or experience. The sun is a representation of consciousness because of the qualities of illumination, life giving, being a neutral presence etc.

[75] Using bīja akṣara-s or seed syllables.

12. In the ancient days, you can see references in the Rāmāyaṇa that Sītā was doing sandhyāvandana. When Hanumān went to find Sītā, the story says that he sought a riverbank as it was evening time and he inferred that she would be near the water in order to practice sandhyāvandana.[76] Similarly, when Rāma goes to see his mother Kausalyā before leaving for exile in the forest, it is said that she was practicing pranayama and meditation.[77]

13. A yajña is to offer an object to the divine or a force[78] with a mantra and a specific intention. In sandhyāvandana, we offer water to the sun with gāyatrī mantra with the intention of our mind becoming clear and awakened.

14. The three key steps are: the symbolic offering of water to the sun, pranayama, and meditation with gāyatrī mantra. If you need to shorten the sandhyāvandana, you must focus on these three steps.

Rejuvenating through ritual

Date: 1977, 1981 | Topic series: Sandhyāvandana, Gheraṇḍa Samhitā

1. To purify any object and renew it, we can see that, in the world outside, we use three steps.

2. The first is the use of air. It dries the object and thereby cleanses it.

3. The second is the use of fire. It heats the object, thereby burning away the impurities inside it.

---

[76] Valmiki Ramayana, Sundara Kanda 14.49

[77] Valmiki Ramayana, Ayodhya Kanda 4.33 & 20.19.

[78] devatā or śakti

4. The third is the use of water. It rejuvenates the object, restoring it.

5. The actions of these three—air, fire, and water—in the external world, change the nature of objects by cleaning, purifying, and rejuvenating, in the world outside.

6. The same process can be done within us. This is part of the ritual of sandhyāvandana too. Through pranayama, we dry the impurities. With gāyatrī mantra repetition, we burn away our old saṃskāra-s. With meditation of the meaning of the mantra, we create a new person.

7. You can do also this in pranayama with seed mantra-s of air, fire, and water. Use the yam sound for drying, as the seed syllable of air. Use the ram sound for heating, as the seed syllable of fire. Use the vam sound for rejuvenation, as the seed syllable of water.

6 / *Ayurveda & Yoga*

In 1981, Krishnamacharya gave a series of lectures on ayurveda, particularly, how ayurveda is connected with yoga, and how these two systems can support each other.

Krishnamacharya was not an ayurvedic physician. However, he did give a deep view into the connection between yoga and ayurveda. Further, he had many experiential insights to share about how we can manage our diet and senses.

He was always insistent on the importance of moderate and healthful food for a yoga practitioner. He used to refer to the Chāndogya Upaniṣad, that food is the foundation of a steady mind. Similarly, he would refer to the Haṭha Yoga Pradīpikā, noting that overeating is the first barrier for a hatha yogi. There is no yoga without "food control," was his firm principle.

Of course, there was never any question of him eating out at a restaurant. He always ate balanced food cooked at home. He used to note that eating excessively sour, spicy, or other such unbalancing foods would damage our health.

Our feelings towards food should be positive. Simple ritual practices he emphasized could help with this. Further, food is a key for both agni and prāṇa.

He used to emphasize that wellbeing and spiritual transformation are out of reach if we do not manage our senses and daily lifestyle. Yoga plays an important role in this.

Why yoga is important, from the view of ayurveda

Date: 1981 | Topic series: Ayurveda and yoga

1. How many diseases exist? They are innumerable. Why? The constituents of the physical world are innumerable and so are their combinations. So, the imbalances that can result are also beyond count. This means that the ways in which these imbalances can be brought back to balance is also innumerable. This is why ayurveda says that herbs that can be medicinal are countless: "There is nothing in this world that is not a medicine."[79]

2. Ayurveda says that disease may result from three causes. The first cause is inappropriate connection between senses and their objects. This happens due to the imbalanced feelings of desire, anger, fear etc. in our mind and senses.

3. The second cause is absence of wisdom and awareness. We do actions that we should not do, that will harm us. We "pay the penalty" for that. The underlying reason is imprudence due to instigation by our senses.

4. The third cause is change. We experience changes in our environment and with seasons. We need to watch over that and make wise choices.

5. We cannot prevent the connection between our senses and their objects. For example, the eyes will always see. We cannot also

---

[79] This is a famous quotation from the Caraka Samhitā (Sūtra Sthāna 26.12): "na anauṣaḍhaṁ jagati kiñcit dravyam upalabhyate" meaning "there is no herb in this world that is not a medicine."

stop change from taking place, in the world outside or in our body.

6. So, the most important of these three is the one that we can control—the second one: absence of wisdom and awareness. We can manage that only by steadying our mind. The way to do that is through yoga. This is why yoga is very important in preventing disease from the view of ayurveda.
7. Agni and prāṇa are always connected. We do stepped breathing in pranayama. We can do the same in Vedic chanting. This will help increase the agni.
8. We need to assess the knowledge and capacity of the person before starting any treatment.

Internal and external cleansing in ayurveda and yoga

Date: 1981 | Topic series: Ayurveda and yoga

1. Both yoga and ayurveda have means for external and internal cleansing of our body.
2. In ayurveda, we purify the body from a more external layer by using oil application, bathing, and exercise. We purify the body from a more internal layer by giving medicines.
3. These steps exist in yoga too. For more external cleansing, we use asana with breathing. For more internal cleansing, we use pranayama.
4. Vedic chanting can also be used in yoga to create internal cleansing. The wellbeing that comes to us from medicines is different from that which comes to us from chanting.

5. Vedic chanting is like an "inner dance." In dance, we must watch each step, each movement. Similarly, in Vedic chanting, we use specific rules to guide and mindfully watch over each step, such as our pronunciation. These rules are explained in the beginning of the Taittiriya Upaniṣad in the Śikṣāvalli.
6. Through proper Vedic chanting, our agni (internal heat, metabolism) increases. This creates inner purification.
7. For medicine to work, agni and digestion should be okay. This is a basic principle in ayurveda. This is why ayurveda emphasizes some medicines to increase the agni.

The six tastes and mental wellbeing

Date: 1981 | Topic series: Ayurveda and yoga

1. The cause for diseases to grow is the food we eat. That food has six tastes. (Sweet, sour, salty, spicy, bitter, astringent according to Ayurveda.)
2. These six tastes affect the six waves of bondage in our mind (desire, anger, greed, delusion, pride, envy).
3. The Chāndogya Upaniṣad (7.26.2) says, "By purity of food, the mind is purified." It is said that 1 out of 16 parts of the food we eat reaches our mind and influences its functioning.
4. The Bhagavad Gita (17.8-10) explains the connection between food and the three guṇa-s. Food that is sweet, pleasing, moist increases sattva. Food that is spicy, sour, salty increases rajas. Food that is tasteless, leftover, and impure increases tamas.
5. By changing our food, we can influence the three doṣa-s, and thereby improve our physical and mental wellbeing.

Prāṇa agni hotra bhāvana: when eating

Date: 1973 | Topic series: Praśna Upaniṣad

In the ancient times, there were formal, large rituals based on the Vedas (called a yāga). The rituals were done for a person (the host) and his wife. The performance required four Vedic experts—one each from the Ṛg Veda, Yajur Veda, Sāma Veda, and Atharva Veda. They had different roles and were given specific titles.

1. These six roles of functions are essential in the major Vedic rituals:

Name	**Role**
Hota	Chants mantras from the Ṛg Veda.
Adhvaryu	Chants mantras from the Yajur Veda
Udgātā	Chants mantras from the Sāma Veda
Bramhā	Chants mantras from the Atharva Veda and supervises the whole ritual.
Patni	Wife
Yajamāna	Host/Doer

2. Food should not be eaten just for taste. It is an offering to the Divine. First, we offer the food to Divine with a yajña (ritual) outside. Then we offer it to the Divine inside us when we eat, using an inner ritual. This ritual is known as prāṇa agni hotra.

3. Just as there are six roles of functions in major Vedic rituals, we should practice bhāvana of all these six within us in this manner:

Role	**Vāyu**
Hota	prāṇa vāyu

Role	Vāyu
Adhvaryu	samāna vāyu
Udgātā	udāna vāyu
Bramhā	vyāna vāyu
Patni	apāna vāyu
Yajamāna	manas (mind)

4. When eating, agni and prāṇa together process the food and distribute it. These vāyus are parts of that process.
5. Yajña is to make an offering to a deity with an intention. Here the deity is prāṇa. We offer food to prāṇa with the intention of nurturing a sāttvic state of mind and body.
6. The mantras used for this are "prāṇaya svāhā, apānaya svāhā" etc. from the Nārāyaṇa Upaniṣad: "May this prāṇa digest my food and be calm and auspicious within me." Similarly, for each of the vāyus.
7. If the prāṇa is to be well-managed, the mind has to actively control it. Hence the mind is yajamāna.
8. Apāna is patni (wife) because the wife helps out with various tasks, supporting. Like that apāna moves upward and reaches the region of the agni, spreading and supporting.
9. The internal bhāvana is also key: we must consume food with the intention that it is an offering to the Divine within.

Yoga and the abdominal organs

Date: 1981 | Topic series: Ayurveda and yoga

1. This topic is related to the explanation of vāta. The Caraka Samhitā speaks about this in the chapter Vātakalākalīya Adhyāya (Sūtrasthana 12).
2. How can we protect the function of vāta and prevent the decline of prāṇa?
3. One of the major reasons for ill-health is obesity. The abdominal organs may be enlarged or out of place.
4. A person who is overweight will not be able to do long inhalation and exhalation. He is unable to take in air deeply from outside.
5. To decrease this enlargement, we must use hold after exhalation. The practice for this is taḍāga-mudrā.
6. The root cause of disease is the taḍāga or "pond"—our abdomen.
7. First, we should teach taḍāga-mudrā. Then we can teach dvipādapīṭham (bridge), followed by ūrdhva-prasṛta-pādāsana (lifting the legs).

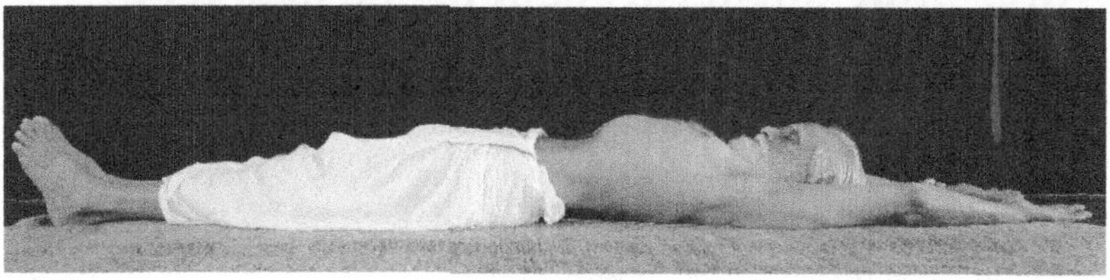

taḍāga-mudrā

For treatments to work well, control vāta with pranayama

Date: 1981 | Topic series: Ayurveda and yoga

1. The Vedas praise vāta, saying, "You are the medicine for the whole world." In our body too, vāta carries the qualities of the other doṣa-s.[80] The Taittirīya Āraṇyaka says that vāta is prāṇa (life force).

2. If vāta is disturbed, we will experience problems like dizziness, vomiting, gas formation, and many other issues.

3. If vāta is excessive, we need to be careful even with surgery. Medicines may also not work well. For treatments to work well, we must first bring vāta under control.

4. By managing our breath, we can keep our vāta in control. For this, pranayama is important.

5. In this context, anuloma-ujjāyī, nāḍīśodhana, and holding after exhalation are especially relevant.

Three attachments in vedanta and ayurveda

Date: 1981 | Topic series: Ayurveda and yoga

1. Vedanta says that we should let go of three attachments to attain freedom (mokṣa): attachment to money, attachment to spouse, and attachment to one's children.[81]

---

[80] This capacity of vāta is given the name *yogavāhī* in ayurveda.

[81] This is termed *īṣaṇā-traya* in Vedanta, meaning *three bindings*.

2. Ayurveda, however, recommends that we must maintain these attachments, but we should watch over them well. Only then will we be well in our normal life.
3. Attachment to prāṇa: take care of your life functions.
4. Attachment to wealth: you need to earn money to provide for your family and yourself. Extreme poverty will result in harm to you and those who depend on you. So, if you have the capacity, you should earn enough to provide the necessities.
5. Attachment to spiritual growth: you must investigate the true nature of your self and devote some time and energy to spiritual transformation. For this, you need to first ensure that you have taken care of prāṇa and have also earned enough to provide for your basic requirements.

Five triads of wellbeing and ill-health

Date: 1981 | Topic series: Ayurveda and yoga

1. Control the triad of:
    a. Tongue—food habits.
    b. Sex—practice bramhacarya to the reasonable extent you can.

       This is why the Upaniṣads speak of tapas (control over food) and brahmacarya.
    c. Eyes—among the senses, the eyes are most important. The eyes draw us outward and trigger the feeling that, "I want this or that." Hence, we have the practice of trāṭaka.
2. Increase the triad of:
    a. Strength of the senses.

   b. Strength of the body.

   c. Strength of the mind.

3. Protect the triad of these locations:

   a. Heart region

   b. Navel

   c. Crown of the head

   These are the locations of the three agni-s.

4. Manage this triad as the source of ill-health:

   a. Mental sources: because we do not get what we want, our mind gets disturbed.

   b. Seasonal sources: because the seasons change, and they impact our health.

   c. Innate sources: the internal imbalance of the doṣa-s.

5. Cultivate this triad as the pillars of energy:

   a. Diet

   b. Sleep

   c. Moderation in sex

What is unsaid and cannot be said in writing

A *guru* is not just an inspiration. Inspiration often only provides a temporary boost to our motivation. From the teaching of a true guru, a strong and lasting conviction should arise in our mind that, "I must do this in my life. This is good for me. This is the path I should follow toward wellbeing and inner peace." A guru should be the reason for important positive transformations in our lives.

Many people even in my family circle asked Indra and me in those days, in the 1970s and 80s, "Why are you studying yoga with Krishnamacharya year after year and spending your time teaching yoga? You are an engineer with a diploma in management, in a good job. Why don't you just pursue this as a career?"

It is not possible to fully understand this unless one experiences the presence of such a guru in their lives. The impact of Krishnamacharya fundamentally transformed the course of not only my life, but that of Indra and my children, Nitya and Ganesh too.

Therefore, as a family, we stayed with him till his demise without wavering, until his last breath—I was one of the few people who carried his mortal remains to the cremation ground.

In turn, he was fully aware of my commitment to him as a disciple, especially as time went on. That is the reason why this book can exist, that these teachings can be passed on now.

Fundamentally, these topics can only be learned from an experienced teacher. Krishnamacharya used to insist on that. He also used to keep cautioning, learn from a sound teacher always.

Yoga is practical. It teaches us life-transformation skills and the knowledge needed for that. It is not a lecture-based system. We need the wisdom of someone who has done it. If we wish to ascend a mountain, only someone who is climbing or has already reached the top can guide another. Theoretical advice from reading about climbing is not enough.

The theory also takes years to deepen. On the first or even second pass, you will understand something, but many aspects will remain vague. Only when you spend time studying, you will slowly understand the connections and insights. For the most part, understanding body, breath, senses, and mind is not about innovating. Nothing significant changed in millennia. The path requires depth and patience.

Much cannot be said in writing alone. For instance, his classes on pranayama, rituals, and Vedic chanting were accompanied by demonstrations and personal guidance. Words on a page cannot convey that, neither can it convey his presence. Therefore, we have selected only a fraction that we can make available.

There are also barriers in experience. He delivered these teachings to me as a personal and long-term student who was in a pathway of years of study with him. The student also has to be ready to receive the teachings. The gap has to be bridged by studies and practice with the teacher. The writings go along with the teachings.

Yoga is a subjective experience, a transformation. As Krishnamacharya would say so many times, yoga will succeed only with the right bhava, the inner experience.

With study and practice, all these teachings become clear. Both knowledge and application are essential.

In this book, we are careful not to bring Krishnamacharya down to our level. We must climb up towards him gradually!

About the authors

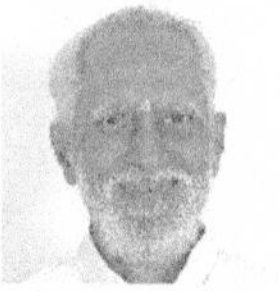

A. G. Mohan is one of the foremost yoga masters in this era. He began his yoga journey in 1971, spending nearly two decades as a personal student of the legendary yogi Sri Krishnamacharya. Then he immersed himself in further wide-ranging studies of ayurveda, sāṃkhya, tantra, ancient India dramatics, jyotiṣa, and more over decades. He is the author of several books on yoga, including *Yoga for Body, Breath, and Mind, Yoga Therapy*, and *Krishnamacharya: His Life and Teachings.*

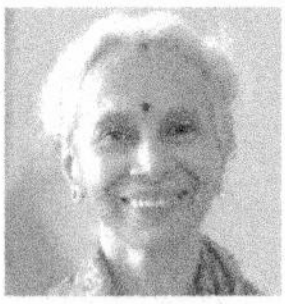

Indra Mohan began her yoga studies along with her husband, A.G. Mohan, in 1971. She is one of few people to receive a post-graduate diploma in yoga from Sri Krishnamacharya. She is appreciated by students not only for her extensive knowledge and clear teachings, but also for her wisdom and calm presence. She has guided many thousands of students over five decades to increase their wellbeing, manage their health problems, and find personal and spiritual transformation.

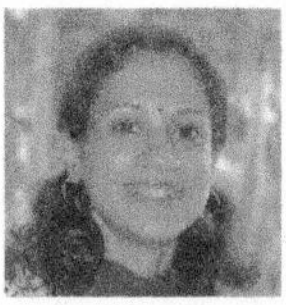

Nitya Mohan, daughter of A. G. Mohan and Indra Mohan, learned yoga from childhood in the tradition of Sri Krishnamacharya. She trained in ancient studies, including Sanskrit and related areas, from a young age. She holds a degree in music and is an exponent of Vedic chanting, having conducted numerous seminars and given concerts internationally. A skilled and experienced teacher, she has been running the Svastha training programs in Singapore for two decades.

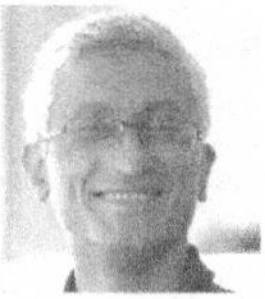

Dr. Ganesh Mohan, son of A. G. Mohan and Indra Mohan, learned yoga from childhood in the tradition of Sri Krishnamacharya. He trained in ancient studies including Sanskrit, Vedic chanting, and Ayurveda and then went on to become a modern medical doctor. He integrates a full spectrum of holistic well-being methods in his work: movement, breathing, meditation and mindfulness, lifestyle, diet, relationships, life guidance and more. He has extensive experience with thousands of students and patients across the world. He directs the the Svastha Yoga Therapy Program. He is the co-author of numerous books published internationally, such as *Yoga Therapy, Krishnamacharya: His Life and Teachings*, and *Yoga Reminder*. With his father, he is the translator of the important Sanskrit yoga texts, *Yoga Yajnavalkya* and *Hatha Yoga Pradipika*.

Made in the USA
Las Vegas, NV
24 August 2023

76560409R00069